ARTEM KUDELIA PHD

Theory & History of Hypnosis

Exploring Altered State of Mind in Trance

First edition

ISBN: 9798853600355

This book was professionally typeset on Reedsy.
Find out more at reedsy.com

Hypnotic trance is a unique psychological state with specific physiological attributes that, at first glance, resemble sleep and are characterized by the individual's behavior under the control of a different state of consciousness, distinct from normal consciousness, defined for convenience as the unconscious or subconscious.

Milton Erickson

Contents

Foreword

The aim of the author of this book is twofold - to acquaint readers with the intricate and profound world of hypnosis and to showcase its "artistry." Until now, hypnosis has been relatively rarely associated with conscientious clinical practice in the eyes of the public and even within certain professional circles. When people hear the word "hypnosis," the first things that come to mind for the so-called "lay psychologist" (and not only for them but also for respectable and successful psychologists with professional education) are "tricks," "deception," "coding," "circus," "charlatanism," and the like. Many individuals are still ensnared by cultural myths about hypnosis that originated during the time of Mesmer.

Meanwhile, the number of psychotherapists, both domestically and abroad, who confidently assert that hypnosis plays a vital role in their professional lives and is a key to success in their work is steadily growing. Numerous practitioners in the field of clinical psychology observe that incorporating suggestive influence as a primary component of intervention leads to profound transformations in clients' thinking, emotions, and behaviors. Some of the beneficial effects of hypnosis encompass "establishing a close collaboration with the client," the ability to "precisely target various motivational, cognitive, or behavioral mechanisms of mental disorders," achieving the "optimal combination of effective intervention strategies and methods," "aligning the client's attitude towards therapy as a whole," and inducing "profound, stable, and long-lasting changes" in personality and psyche, among others.

The presented book can prove highly valuable for both professionals and newcomers. Professionals have the opportunity to systematize and organize their existing knowledge about fundamental trance phenomena (the authors describe approximately forty phenomena), their manifestations, and their utilization in psychotherapeutic practice. Readers receive this invaluable information firsthand: the authors generously share their own experiences as well as examples from the practices of renowned domestic and international specialists (A. Danilov, V. Raikov, R. Bandler, S. Gilligan, L. Le Cron, B. Hellinger, M. Erickson, etc.). The authors are convinced that virtually any trance phenomenon can be utilized as a metaphor for transformation. To achieve this, they have developed a step-by-step model for utilizing hypnotic phenomena in psychotherapy.

For newcomers, this book can serve as a guide for embarking on their journey. The most significant aspect in which this guide can assist novice hypnotherapists is by relieving them of the fear and apprehension that they might "do hypnosis wrong."

The goal of the authors of this book is twofold - to acquaint readers with the complex and rich world of hypnosis and to showcase its "artistry." Until now, in the eyes of the public and even in certain professional circles, hypnosis has been relatively rarely associated with conscientious clinical practice. The first things that come to mind for the so-called "lay psychologist" (and not only for them, but also for respectable and successful practicing psychologists with professional education) in relation to this word are "tricks," "deception," "coding," "circus," "charlatanism," and so on. Many are still trapped in cultural myths about hypnosis that originated in the time of Mesmer.

Meanwhile, the number of psychotherapists, both abroad and in our country, who confidently assert that hypnosis plays an important role in their professional lives and is a guarantee of success in their work is steadily increasing. Many representatives of clinical practice note that the inclusion of suggestive influence as a primary component of intervention contributes to profound transformations in clients' thinking, emotions, and actions. Among the beneficial effects of hypnosis are the "achievement of close collaboration with the client," the possibility to "precisely target specific motivational, cognitive, or behavioral mechanisms of psychological disorders," to achieve the "best combination of effective intervention strategies and methods," to "prepare the client for therapy as a whole," and to induce "deep, stable, and long-lasting changes" in personality and psyche, from the cognitive to the behavioral level.

The proposed book can be highly useful for both professionals and beginners. The former have the opportunity to systematize and organize their existing knowledge about basic trance phenomena (the authors describe about forty phenomena), their manifestations, and their use in psychotherapeutic practice. This valuable information is presented firsthand: the authors generously share their own experience as well as examples from the practice of well-known domestic and foreign specialists (R. Bandler, S. Gilligan, L. Lechron, B. Hellinger, M. Erickson, A. Danilov, V. Raikov etc.). The authors are convinced that essentially any trance phenomenon can be used as a metaphor for transformation. To this end, they have developed a step-by-step model for the use of hypnotic phenomena in psychotherapy.

For beginners, this book can serve as a guide to "getting started." The main reason that this guide can be beneficial for aspiring hypnotherapists is that it dispels their fear and concerns about "doing hypnosis incorrectly."

The book allows readers to obtain a comprehensive understanding of the history of hypnotherapy, the theoretical concepts underlying hypnosis, and the practical issues that arise when attempting to induce trance. By mastering this captivating text, the discerning reader, striving for excellence, can successfully acquire the essential skills of using hypnosis in psychotherapy. The authors have taken care of readers who aspire not only to know but also to be able to "move from words to action," to test the effectiveness of various hypnotic phenomena. For this purpose, step-by-step algorithms of trance work are provided, encompassing the procedural experience of both international and the authors' own extensive years of psychotherapeutic practice.

The system of beliefs and practices underlying the concept of "depth of hypnotic trance" has been significantly organized. Paying careful attention to the legacy of A. Forel and, unfortunately, the often-forgotten talented physiologist and hypnotist E. Katkov from Kharkov, the authors have developed and substantiated a practical multi-level model (consisting of 12 levels) of the hypnotic trance.

Like any good and seemingly purely practical manual, the work of A. S. Kudelia stimulates the reader's reflections on scientific and research topics. Most of these topics revolve around three fundamental directions.

Firstly, there is the problem of seeking rigorous experimental evidence of the effectiveness of psychotherapy (i.e., ensuring the empirical basis of psychotherapy). Inducing trance (or, conversely, refraining from inducing it) can be used as a means of varying the independent variable, enabling confident statements about causal relationships in the process of psychotherapeutic interventions.

Secondly, it is the emergence of additional impetus in memory research (episodic, implicit, emotional, motor, etc.). The issue of memory has long been and still remains relevant for the Kharkiv psychological school. It is worth mentioning that both authors are from Kharkov and are therefore representatives of this scientific school. Their perspective on the manifestations and resources of memory is analyzed in connection with the problem of repressed memories and providing elegant access to them in the process of trance work.

Thirdly, it is the interconnection between the authors' practical developments in the field of hypnotherapy and the achievements of cognitive neuroscience. These advancements have become possible in recent times due to the development of state-of-the-art brain activity visualization techniques, including functional magnetic resonance imaging (fMRI). The authors seek to answer not only the question of what hypnosis is from a psychological perspective but also the question of its physiological mechanisms.

While acquainting oneself with this guide, even the most skeptical reader of hypnosis becomes filled with optimism. The authors are highly persuasive in their arguments when they demonstrate that a psychotherapist can use any potential that a client possesses. Any response that the client provides in any specific situation, including their own symptoms, can be utilized. The book is filled with significant didactic material, making it an indispensable manual, especially for psychology and medical students interested in mastering not only the art of hypnotherapy but also achieving excellence in psychotherapy as a whole.

Preface

In the modern world, hypnotic suggestion has a multifaceted context of implementation. Hypnosis is familiar to many people who are not involved with it in a professional context and primarily understand it through social myths that abound in society. This book will be devoted to a comprehensive description of the process of hypnosis, with a particular focus on the psychotherapeutic context and working with trance in patients who require psychotherapeutic assistance. We will cover the psychological, physiological, cultural, and social aspects that provide an opportunity to view hypnosis as a mysterious and mystical process, a philosophy, and a neuro-chemical process in the human brain, as well as a socio-cultural phenomenon rooted in all psycho-spiritual traditions of the world.

Therefore, one of the emphases of this work will be an anthropological context, narrating the history of the formation of conceptions of hypnosis in various parts of the world and how this psycho-spiritual phenomenon became part of the practice of modern medicine in psychiatry, psychotherapy, and surgical anesthesia. What exactly is hypnosis from the perspective of psychology and physiology? What is the correct definition of such a process? Where can this phenomenon be applied in a social context? What personal characteristics of an individual will determine their ability to enter the state of hypnosis quickly or slowly, deeply or superficially? What can facilitate or hinder the induction of hypnosis? What knowledge and skills are necessary for a hypnotherapist to create hypnotic induction and interact with the patient in a trance state? We will seek answers to these questions in this book.

A part of the work will be devoted to general cognitive information, while another part will focus on the description of direct methods and techniques for inducing hypnosis. By mastering these techniques, you will be able to acquire a basic level of proficiency in the practice of hypnosis. It is better to practice other examples in training groups, as there are many nuances that are difficult to convey through text alone, and real demonstrations and trainer comments are necessary in the process of training work.

The communicative aspect of hypnosis can extend beyond the psychotherapeutic context, where we can discover that at a deeper level, hypnosis techniques are simply advanced forms of communication related to emotional intelligence, which is an integral part of the human experience and the ability to change one's own states and the states of others. To some extent, inducing trance is the ability to effectively convey information to another person. It is a tool that is not inherently moral, and depending on whose hands it falls into, it can heal or harm.

Therefore, a part of the work will be dedicated to discussing how people, even those unfamiliar with the phenomenon of hypnosis, regularly apply it in their communication, often creating non-ecological states in their interlocutors. Stage hypnosis, as one of the entertainment contexts, is highly con-troversial and also not very ecological, and it will also be part of our discussion, where we will touch upon the main strategies used by stage hypnotists. Essentially, their methods and the methods of psychotherapeutic hypnosis have a common root, but the techniques, practices, and phenomenology of trance can significantly differ.

Many individuals involved in mysticism and occultism apply a large number of hypnotic practices, where they perceive and define hypnotic phenomena as supernatural, magical manifestations. We will not discuss all of these situations in general, but a significant part of such phenomena can be recreated by an individual with hypnosis skills through fairly simple procedures. We will discuss and explore all of these topics throughout the book. For starters, let's begin with the history of the formation of conceptions of altered states of perception, hypnosis, trance, and various practices that have helped achieve them at different times.

Acknowledgement

I would like to express our gratitude to my teachers in the field of psychotherapy and hypnotherapy: Betty Erickson, Stephen Gilligan, Jean Becchio, and Claude Viro. I would also like to thank the students and patients who participated in scientific and psychotherapeutic research, as well as all the individuals who have contributed in various ways to the creation of this book.

BONUS: Your Free Gifts

Use QR code or link psychemaster.com/psychology-and-psychotherapy-books-series to **receive a free eBook "Psychotherapy Introduction"** from the author, plus links to online **psychological tests** and quizzes.

These resources will guide you in evaluating your well-being and deciding whether to consult a **mental health professional**. You can complete each test in under five minutes and receive immediate results.

1

History of Trance Practices and Hypnotherapy

At this very place, by the throne, resides the beautiful and youthful god of sleep, Hypnos. Noiselessly, he soars above the earth on his wings, holding poppy heads in his hands and pouring a soporific elixir from his horn. With his wondrous wand, he gently touches the eyes of humans, softly closing their lids and immersing mortals in a sweet slumber. Mighty is the god Hypnos, against whom neither mortals nor gods nor even the thunderer Zeus can resist. Hypnos closes his eyes as well, plunging him into a deep sleep.

  Myths of ancient Greece

If we consider the historical perspective, the phenomenon of trance induction and self-induced trance has existed throughout the entire existence of rational human beings. The presence of the social role of a shaman within a group, a person who assumed multifaceted functions as a philosopher, educator, and healer, has been consistent.

Modern anthropology indicates that the history of shamanism dates back 40,000 to 60,000 years, from the early stages of the shamanic role to its later manifestations in contemporary activities. Archaic shamanism played a multifaceted and socially significant role, complementing the role of a leader dominant in external social aspects of governance. The shaman took on the role of explaining, often, the inexplicable, the unseen, and the unknown, which could now be termed spiritual or numinous.

Mapping reality, giving names to the inexplicable, attempting to understand the structure of the universe and its governing principles—shamanism largely anticipated religion, being more of a pre-religion, a philosophy as an aspect of life wisdom, and an empirical criterion for understanding the world.

The shaman is a person standing on the border between the

living and the dead, between the realm of the conscious and the realm of dreams, between the apparent and the unseen, between the comprehensible and the incomprehensible. The shaman serves as a connecting link between the concepts of duality within the human mind, accustomed to dividing everything into good and bad, white and black, understandable and incomprehensible. This is precisely what defines the fundamental difference between humans and animals—their reasoning, which, in the overwhelming majority of cases, is unburdened by concepts of morality and duality.

Where there is morality, there is duality, and naturally, a latent sense arises to return to a feeling of wholeness and connection. Mapping reality primarily served as a natural psychotherapeutic function in ancient tribes because when you understand, or think you understand, the world, the level of anxious reactions naturally decreases. Every time we give something a name, we gain a sense of control. However, mapping is merely the first step, followed by the creation of a significant number of practices, patterns, and forms of activity with a specific goal: to interact with the unseen, the incomprehensible, and the unknown.

Creation of rituals whose essence was to induce altered states of consciousness aimed at solving pressing problems: emotional, physical, social, peaceful, military, agrarian, and so on. This is where we begin to recognize the fundamental roots of hypnotic influence and the fact that the intention behind modern clinical psychotherapeutic or anesthesiological hypnosis bears little difference from ancient archaic forms of shamanic chanting and dancing.

These traditions date back thousands or even tens of thousands of years, each with its own history, phenomenology, cul-

3

ture, and interpretation of reality. While there are differences in the details, the abstract cores of shamanic traditions are similar, possessing almost identical essences. The variations lie in the accents.

Without delving into a detailed historical exploration of shamanism, let us limit ourselves to understanding this form of activity as the origin, archetype, and primal form of the shaman—a transceiver capable of embodying multiple hypostases, external social roles, as well as internal numinous experiences accessible primarily to the individual rather than the crowd.

The ritualized process of altering states carries another crucial aspect—sublimation and ennoblement. In ancient Hinduism, the ability to perform ritual psychospiritual rites was a priority for the Brahmins, a caste of scholars and priests who considered this privilege one of the main criteria that defined a person's humanity. In other words, the ability to perform rituals aimed at altering consciousness, both in others and in oneself, and through these altered states, gain access to knowledge, skills, healing, and new conceptions of the world.

An important conclusion that can be drawn from these findings is that the primal prototype of the trans-like, hypnotic suggestor can play a crucial and prevailing role in the evolutionary process, both at the social group and intrapersonal levels. In subsequent chapters of our book, we will revisit how the trance process influences learning and the restoration of healthy mental and somatic homeostasis in individuals. For now, let us direct our attention to its more social and archaic aspects.

Beyond basic needs such as food, sex is also a fundamental aspect of human personality. If we carefully analyze various

4

types of activities in ancient and modern humans, ranging from highly intellectual individuals to simpler ones, from young to elderly, we will discover that in every person's life, there are tools for altering states of consciousness that manifest in sublimated and non-sublimated forms. In other words, sex, sleep, and indulging in delicious food are natural instruments for altering states of consciousness.

However, the moment a person discovers substitutes for instinctual trance forms of activity, their personality undergoes radical changes, becoming more complex due to increased values and beliefs and the alteration of the value-motivational hierarchy. Aggression and excessive eroticism, which were more characteristic of ancient humans, gradually gave way to other forms of activity. Complete replacement only occurs in a few individuals, often those associated with shamanic or other psychospiritual orientations.

We can also observe that the abandonment of instinctual trance for specific periods of time in many spiritual cultures is primarily an initiatory act, where the adept renounces the animal in favor of the numinous to acquire personal strength, self-control, willpower, and the ability to face life's difficulties, undergoing significant social transformations.

The trans-like hypnotic process allows individuals to train their volitional qualities, such as volition, goal-setting, and decision-making, and it enhances the activity of the prefrontal lobes of the brain's cerebral hemispheres, as understood in modern neurophysiology. However, it is worth noting that it is the sublimating trance that leads to the latter.

In shamanism, the process of acquiring volitional qualities was equated with the process of gaining personal power, enabling individuals to live their lives, fulfill their social roles, and fulfill their destinies more effectively. The sacralization of trance as an evolutionary social and personal process can be traced as a structural element in all psycho-spiritual systems in the world.

Hypnosis, on the other hand, in a more contemporary sense, is merely a modern variation of shamanic rituals, oriented towards a more scientifically objective perception of the world, unlike the mythic worldview of ancient shamans. Naturally, we can see a wide range of differences when discussing pre-rational, rational, and post-rational ways of mapping reality.

Many modern scientists may not take shamanism and the psycho-practices of religion seriously, often dismissing them as unrealistic metaphorical descriptions of reality. However, once we begin to examine the structure of the experience, both ancient and modern, everything falls into place. The structure is almost identical, pursuing nearly identical goals and serving as the progenitor, the "genetic code," which determines the development of its "successor."

Religions can be viewed as the next stage of development in trance-hypnotic techniques, where the internal psychogeography of states is fundamentally transformed and ordered, which can be recreated through trance induction. A more consolidated and predominantly monotheistic form of perceiving archetypes of the unconscious is formed, naturally beginning to transform not only the maps of reality and the ritual practices of interaction with them but also the social fabric of human relationships in society.

The gradual transformation of shamanism into religious movements began to change the value-motivational structure of trance practices, tantric practices, psychospiritual visualizations, somatic practices, attentional fixations, and

6

various types of meditations, leading to altered states of consciousness. However, the structure of the trance process itself remains unchanged from ancient shamanism to modern hypnotic psychotherapy. The social roles that utilize trance undergo transformation and modification. To some extent, it can be said that the type of trance induction within a social group largely determines an individual's social, ethnic, and moral orientation. For example, a Christian priest may disapprove of the work of a hypnotherapist, stating that "hypnosis steals the soul," an Islamic imam may criticize Hatha yoga as a practice of the infidels, and a scientific psychotherapist may skeptically regard transcendental meditation, considering it unscientific. Of course, it is an exaggeration to claim that all individuals with a particular psychospiritual orientation will necessarily avoid the trance-hypnotic methods of other schools. Nonetheless, there are integrative personalities that attempt to combine a multitude of different practices in their activities.

When examining the history of religion, we discover that various religious schools have been known to adopt certain practices from others throughout the centuries and present them as their own. However, currently, most canonized psychospiritual institutions, at a formal level, refrain from adopting practices from other schools. A psychotherapist in a clinic who treats patients through prayer and chanting mantras would likely be seen as overly eccentric. Similarly, a priest who attempts to conduct Ericksonian hypnotherapy during a church service may face suspension from their duties.

The preferred type of trance state determines the personal identity of an individual, along with the beliefs and values they embody. Consequently, the trance experience of one's own group is usually perceived as good and right, while the trance of another group is often seen as evil, until the individual reaches more integrative levels of identity development. Unfortunately, such occurrences are rare.

Trance-hypnotic practice has not always been exclusively associated with shamanic and religious contexts. Individuals involved in various other activities have, do, and will continue to enter hypnotic trance states that differ in quality from shamanic, religious, and psychotherapeutic trance states. These individuals may include hunters, athletes, warriors, and others.

It is enough to recall the hunter in archaic times who would draw an image of a bison on the ground or on a rock, symbolically slaying it with a spear to ensure a successful hunt.

The Scandinavian berserker warrior enters a state of combat trance, in which their physical strength significantly increases and their ability to feel pain diminishes.

The ancient Greek runner, capable of running over 200 kilometers without stopping from one city to another to deliver a message, did not feel fatigue; he was consumed by the rhythm of running.

While we can provide more historical examples, we only formally know about them through history. Let's focus on modern examples of trance masters recorded by contemporary scientists.

A living Dutchman, Wim Hof, demonstrated his ability to stay in icy water for over 2 hours thanks to a self-invented breathing technique. He did this in a laboratory under the supervision of scientists who monitored his body temperature with sensors. It turned out that his body maintained a temperature of 37 degrees Celsius throughout the entire period. Without self-induced trance, such a phenomenon would simply be impossible to replicate.

Ultramarathon runner Dean Karnazes covered 221 kilometers in 24 hours of continuous running. Without the ability to shift and maintain his consciousness in a trance state, this would be utterly unrealistic.

Dutchman Arnold Henske (known as Mirin Dajo) repeatedly demonstrated to doctors in a clinic how he could safely pierce his body with various types of cold weapons.

These are just three examples, and numerous others can be found. Some may appear quite realistic, while others may seem entirely unreal. We assert that all such phenomena are possible and can only be created through self-hypnotic induction.

At times, we encounter natural phenomena that arise spontaneously in individuals or due to specific stressful situations in life. Alternatively, we find that these individuals undergo specialized training to demonstrate such trance phenomena.

The formal starting point for clinical hypnosis can be considered the German physician and healer Franz Anton Mesmer, who developed the doctrine of "animal magnetism."

Franz Anton Mesmer (1734–1815)

Practicing magnet therapy, Mesmer wrote a treatise called "Introductio ad utilem usum Magnetis ex chalybe." Initially, his method involved applying magnets to the patient's body and creating iron-based preparations that were later given to the patients. In describing a case of his therapy, Mesmer writes that the disease left his patient within a few hours. From that moment on, he considers himself the discoverer of a new therapeutic method and continues his research. Later, Mesmer discovers that he himself is capable of "magnetizing" paper, glass, and water and declares that the use of magnets is optional. He sends messages about his discovery to major European universities but receives only doubts about the truthfulness of his discovery in the responses he receives. Mesmer faces an extremely cold reception from the scientific community. In anonymous correspondence from Vienna, he receives critical reviews and even ridicule for his method. After some time being pursued by the German scientific community, Mesmer moves to Paris in 1778.

According to historical accounts, Mesmer's group therapy appeared quite extravagant. Groups of patients were treated by immersing their feet in a fountain with magnetized water. They held onto wires connected to "magnetized" trees with their hands. Mesmer himself accompanied this process on the piano or glass harmonica.

Soon, the French medical community declares war on Mesmer, and he and his methods become the subject of examination by a scientific commission.

The scientific commission concludes that all therapeutic phenomena that could accompany his work method were nothing more than the vivid imagination of the patients. Despite the criticism from the scientific community, Mesmer managed to create his own community called the "Society of Universal Harmony," which had up to 430 members. Additionally, through his therapeutic and social activities, Mesmer manages to amass a considerable fortune, making him one of the wealthiest scientists in Europe.

Mesmer's theory states that disease in a person arises from the uneven distribution of magnetic fluid in the patient's body. He claimed that a doctor could transfer fluid to the patient through magnetic passes or touch.

Mesmer believed that in a state of magnetic trance, patients were capable of foreseeing the future or revealing distant past events, diagnosing diseases, and finding ways to treat them. Despite the highly psychospiritual connotations of his professional pursuits, he believed that the effects he achieved through his methods primarily had a physiological rather than psychological nature.

Despite the criticism of Mesmer's activities, his work continued to be of interest to some scientists, such as D. Braid, I. Bernheim, A. Liebeault, and J.-M. Charcot, for a significant period of time and largely shaped the initial understanding of hypnosis as a clinical practice method.

It was precisely after the establishment of Mesmer's theory in the early 19th century that the practitioners of hypnosis became divided into two key schools:

1. **Fluidists** - followers of Mesmer who believed that the basis of hypnotic suggestion lay in the transmission of magnetic fluids from the magnetizer to the magnetized subject.

2. **Animists** - opponents of Mesmer who believed that no such fluids existed and that the basis of magnetization and hypnotization of the patient was suggestion or imagination.

Although Mesmer did not create the term "magnetism" himself but borrowed it from Paracelsus - Philippus Aureolus Theophrastus Bombastus von Hohenheim (1493–1541), who mainly dealt with medicine and alchemy and did not apply magnetic force as Mesmer did.

Paracelsus

Paracelsus, as far as we know, was the first physician to attempt to explain magnetic phenomena and, in fact, introduced the term itself from the Phoenician language, which meant "that which is transferred to another." Paracelsus hypothesized that magnets could attract not only metallic objects but also disease. He was also one of the first physicians to apply the future-discovered "placebo" effect in his practice. He believed that the power lay not so much in the magnet itself as in the deep belief that a miracle would occur. And it didn't matter what lay behind it.

Independent of Anton Mesmer, a variation of magnetic suggestion was developed in Portugal by Abbé Faria, who later became the prototype of one of the characters in the book "The Count of Monte Cristo." It is not possible to ascertain with certainty whether his method was independently created or borrowed from Mesmer or another person.

The fact is that Faria employed the techniques of fixed gaze, eye-to-eye contact, and verbal suggestion to induce a hypnotic state through repeated words like "you sleep, you fall asleep." Faria's technique shared similarities with the techniques employed by Mesmer and his followers. For example, Faria could take a Christian cross, raise it above another person's head, and ask them to gaze intently at its shining surface, expecting the mesmerized individual to fall asleep.

One of the most interesting successors of Anton Mesmer was the Scottish physician James Braid (1795–1860). While his primary specialization was surgery, at a certain stage of his professional journey, Braid made several discoveries that slightly diverted him from the path of an ordinary surgeon. For instance, he made the intriguing discovery that prolonged fixation on shiny objects could induce a specific, cord-like state in a person.

James Braid (1795–1860)

Having read extensively about Anton Mesmer and the activities of mesmerists, James Braid developed a highly critical attitude towards their practices, considering the phenomenon of magnetism as deception, fraud, and trickery. History reveals interesting facts about James Braid's life. On November 13, 1841, Braid attended a performance by the mesmerist Lafontaine, further convincing himself that what was happening on stage was likely deceit and pretense. To definitively expose Lafontaine, six days later, Braid attended another performance but encountered a phenomenon that would later be termed "eyelid catalepsy." Lafontaine magnetized one of the spectators, suggesting that he was unable to raise his eyelids. And indeed, the "magnetized" subject was unable to lift his eyelids, no matter how hard he tried. This shocked Braid, prompting him to conduct experiments on the application of magnetism within his family and circle of friends.

During one such gathering, Braid asked his friend Walker to fix his gaze on the neck of an empty wine bottle. Braid then lifted the bottle above Walker's eyes to tire them, and after a few minutes, he observed that Walker's eyes closed, his head slightly leaned to the side, and his breathing deepened. Continuing his experiments, Braid focused on fixing the gaze of his subjects on various objects and discovered that he could almost always achieve a similar cord-like effect. He termed this state "nervous sleep." Based on his observations, he concluded that he was dealing not with magnetic force but rather with specific nervous processes occurring in individuals under certain conditions. After some time, Braid found a more suitable name for this phenomenon, in his opinion: "hypnosis," which later became established in the field of science.

One of the notable followers of James Braid's theories was the French physician Hippolyte Bernheim, a professor at the University of Strasbourg. After the Franco-Prussian War of

1871, he relocated to Nancy, where he assumed a position as a clinic professor. There, he established his psychoneurological clinic and began practicing hypnosis for therapeutic and research purposes.

Hippolyte Bernheim (1840–1919)

In many ways, Hippolyte Bernheim's theory related to comparing the hypnotic state to a cord-like phenomenon, viewing it as a kind of variation of sleep. It was Bernheim who first applied hypnosis as therapy in full clinical conditions. He conducted research on hysteria and its connection to hypnotic suggestion phenomena and discovered the phenomenon of hyper suggestibility in hysterical individuals within a clinical context. This led him to consider hysteria and hysterical behavior as manifestations of autosuggestion. Bernheim embarked on the path of a pioneer, unearthing invaluable information that would become key to the art of profiling individuals. Based on a patient's personality profile, he could predict the depth of the hypnotic state, the trance phenomena achievable during hypnosis, and the potential outcomes attainable using hypnotic methods.

One of Bernheim's scientific colleagues in the field of hypnosis research was the French physician Ambroise-Auguste Liébeault (1823–1904). Liébeault was the founder of the "Nancy School" of hypnosis, where he and his colleague Hippolyte Bernheim conducted psychotherapeutic hypnotherapy for patients in their clinic, primarily focusing on hysterical patients. Some sources even attribute him as the father of hypnotherapy, although this claim is somewhat debatable considering the work of figures such as Franz Mesmer, who simply did not use the term "hypnosis" to describe his practices. Naturally, James Braid, who extensively experimented with hypnosis but did not transform it into a widely adopted therapeutic method in clinical conditions, also influenced the field.

The fundamental idea of the Nancy School was that hypnosis itself had nothing to do with animal magnetism or the transmission of magnetic fluids to the patient. Instead, it was directly related to induced suggestion, which actualized the diverse range of hypnotic phenomena.

A. Liébeault had a friendship with Étienne Eugène Azam (1822–1899), the main French disciple of James Braid in France. This association significantly influenced Liébeault's hypnotic practice, aligning it with Braid's theory. Liébeault's primary work in the field of hypnosis was his book "Sleep and its Analogs, Mainly Considered from the Perspective of the Mind's Influence on the Body."

Additionally, Liébeault was greatly influenced by the ideas of Abbé Faria (1746–1819) and Alexandre Jacques François Bertrand (1795–1831).

Thanks to A. A. Liébeault, Sigmund Freud and Émile Coué were drawn to the Nancy School during their time there. Jean-Martin Charcot (1825–1893), the French physician, psychiatrist, and specialist in neurological diseases mentioned in the history of psychiatry as Sigmund Freud's teacher, was one of the most prominent clinical researchers of hypnosis in his clinical practice.

Jean-Martin Charcot (1825–1893)

Jean-Martin Charcot worked at the Salpêtrière Hospital, where he became the chief physician in 1862 and took charge of the department for "non-psychotic epileptics and hysterics." It is worth noting that at that time, hysteria was considered a neurological rather than a psychiatric disorder.

At the beginning of his clinical practice, J.M. Charcot focused primarily on the study and treatment of internal diseases such as tuberculosis, rheumatism, pneumonia, and others. Later, he redirected his interest towards diseases related to brain dysfunction, initiating studies on its structure and the localization of its functions.

While working with hysterical women in the clinic, J.M. Charcot initially believed that hysteria was exclusively a female condition associated with uterine dysfunction. However, during his work with hysterical patients, he discovered that they often suffered from somatic disorders such as blindness, paralysis, and convulsions without exhibiting the typical brain lesions associated with these conditions. Naturally, he also observed that hysterical patients were highly susceptible to hypnotic suggestion. J.-M. Charcot conducted numerous experiments involving the induction of paralysis in various body parts and achieved remarkable success both in creating these conditions and subsequently curing them.

As a result, J.-M. Charcot concluded that during hysteria, a person enters a state akin to hypnosis. It was Charcot who began to refer to hysterical disorder as a natural form of hypnosis since the phenomenology of hysteria and hypnosis were almost entirely identical, with the exception that hysterical patients did not require a hypnotist to induce an altered state of consciousness.

After J.-M. Charcot's death in 1899, his book "The Healing Faith" was published, emphasizing the role of faith as a key factor in the healing process. J.M. Charcot summarized various cases of miraculous healing associated with different spiritual symbols, connecting faith's influence to human neurophysiology. "The healing faith, whether religious or secular, cannot be dichotomous; it is the same cerebral process that produces identical effects," stated J.-M. Charcot. According to him, the patient's firm belief in the healing factor of therapeutic actions becomes a crucial element in the healing process, and the main task of the physician is to instill such conviction in the patient.

Doctors from Nancy adhered to the theory of understanding hypnosis as a general property of suggestibility that manifests in varying intensities. They emphasized its psychological nature, contrasting with J.-M. Charcot, who considered it organic.

Nowadays, it can be confidently stated that both schools were correct and that hypnosis involves both psychological and physiological factors.

Sigmund Freud's interaction with J.-M. Charcot predetermined his professional development and establishment. Freud interned under J.-M. Charcot for four months in 1885. Later, Freud wrote about J.-M. Charcot: "No man has had such an influence on me... I used to leave his lectures with a feeling as if I were leaving Notre-Dame de Paris, full of new insights into perfection."

In the late 19th and early 20th centuries, physicians increasingly sought physiological and scientific justifications for hypnotic processes. Active experimental investigations unfolded in Europe and Russia. For example, in 1881, doctors from Odessa, O.O. Mochutkovsky and B.A. Oks, conducted numerous hypnotic experiments with hysterical patients in the clinic, reproducing phenomena such as paresis, paralysis, catalepsy of the whole body, and multiple personality manifestations.

V.Ya. Danilevsky from Kharkov delivered a report at the International Congress of Physiological Psychology in 1889, discussing experiments on hypnotizing crustaceans, birds, rabbits, and other animals. He concluded that the phenomenon of hypnosis is not exclusive to human beings. It is worth noting that V.M. Bekhterev later conducted experiments on animal hypnosis.

Another psychiatrist, psychoneurologist, and hypnotherapist worth mentioning is Konstantin Ivanovich Platonov (1877–1969), who worked in Kharkov and was a student of V.M. Bekhterev.

Konstantin Ivanovich Platonov (1877–1969)

K.I. Platonov significantly interpreted the processes occurring in a patient during the state of hypnosis as specific neuro-physiological mechanisms. He concluded that the depth of the hypnotic state and, at the same time, the phenomenon of suggestibility in individuals were not necessarily a result of deep hypnotization.

Platonov is also known for his original methodology for pain relief during childbirth and is the author of the 1930 monograph "Speech as a Physiological and Therapeutic Factor" (1930). As mentioned earlier, Sigmund Freud (1856–1939) studied hypnotic suggestion in the Salpêtrière and Nancy schools. At the beginning of his practice, he actively used hypnosis with his patients to recover lost memories of early childhood. In other words, he conducted hypnotic regression to access repressed emotions and facilitate their abreaction (emotional release).

Sigmund Freud (1856–1939)

Most often, he employed the methods of J.-M. Charcot, press-ing his hand against the patient's forehead and inducing sleep, during which the patient was supposed to recall material necessary for therapy. He closely collaborated with his col-league, physician Josef Breuer, who also practiced hypnosis with his patients. Together with J. Breuer, he published the work "Studies on Hysteria." This work became the seminal text for future developments in hypnoanalysis and regression hypnotherapy.

One of J. Breuer's cases with one of his patients became a catalyst for S. Freud's creation of an alternative method of treatment apart from hypnosis. This case is mentioned in psychoanalytic literature under the name "the case of Anna O."

Anna O. was one of J. Breuer's young patients suffering from hysteria, manifested in symptoms such as hysterical paralysis, paresis of the right side of the face, and temporary dissociation of personality. It was revealed that the hysterical symptoms in Anna O. began after she had cared for her bedridden, debilitated father for over two years. J. Breuer worked with Anna for several months, almost every day, sometimes twice a day. He regularly recorded her delusions during her altered states of consciousness and conducted hypnotic sessions with her. He came up with the idea of transcribing what the patient said during her delusions and then reading the same text back to her while inducing her into a hypnotic state. Through this technique, he discovered that after the reading, the patient would start displaying a significant number of emotional ab-reactions. In other words, she would begin to experience intense emotions, cry, scream, and release suppressed emotions during the process of treating her father. J. Breuer continued his experiments with Anna, but after some time, he encountered a significant problem: the patient developed a rare phenomenon called phantom pregnancy, which sometimes occurs in women with hysterical symptoms. When asked about her condition, Anna claimed that she was carrying J. Breuer's baby in her abdomen. After this incident, J. Breuer discontinued the therapy and left with his wife for the Alps, presumably to save their marriage. Breuer named his form of therapy "cathartic therapy," which did not directly evolve into a separate approach but, as a concept and idea, became rooted in numerous future directions of psychotherapeutic practice.

After some time, S. Freud abandoned the practice of hypnosis, which, in his opinion, did not possess sufficient therapeutic depth, in favor of the psychoanalytic method he was developing, based on the technique of free association. Although much later, after the establishment of psychoanalysis, S. Freud hypothesized that pure psychoanalysis could be combined with hypnoanalysis to shorten the duration of therapeutic work, he believed that it might weaken the outcome. His opinion on this matter remains debatable, but unfortunately, his conclusions are unlikely to undergo thorough empirical analysis.

A notable opponent of S. Freud's theories but also a colleague in the practice of hypnotic suggestion, was French psychologist, neuropathologist, and psychiatrist Pierre Marie Félix Janet (1859–1947). Like Freud, he was a student of Jean-Martin Charcot. In his clinical practice, P. Janet developed the "psychological conception of neuroses" and considered neurotic disorders as processes that disrupt the balance between higher and lower mental functions. His theories shared similarities with those of American behaviorists. He believed that consciousness should be regarded "as a special form of act, surpassing elementary behavior" and that psychology should be "objective in the sense that its subject matter should be directly observable." It is also worth noting that P. Janet considered the psychological factor to be the primary influential factor in hypnosis, rather than the physiological factor. According to his perspective, the psychological factor played a fundamental conditioning role in the process of hypnotization.

Pierre Marie Félix Janet (1859–1947)

There are intriguing examples of Pierre Janet's hypnotic work that are worth mentioning. One such case involved a twenty-year-old woman suffering from severe menstrual pain that would begin a few days before her period and continue for several days. Janet employed hypnoanalysis to uncover the cause of the woman's past pain. While in a hypnotic state, she recalled a situation when she was thirteen years old and had just started menstruating. Unaware of what was happening to her, she ventured out into the freezing cold and immersed herself in a barrel of icy water in an attempt to stop the bleeding. Afterward, her menstrual cycle ceased and did not resume until she turned fifteen, but when it returned, it was accompanied by excruciating pain. It should be noted that the reduction or temporary cessation of menstruation can indeed be achieved if a woman immerses herself in icy water during her period. In our own practice, we have encountered several similar cases. However, in our observations, this did not lead to their prolonged cessation as it did in Janet's patient.

After obtaining the analytical material, Janet decided to embark on an unusual experiment with his patient, which he would later refer to as "lying therapy." Janet regressed the patient back to the age of thirteen using hypnoanalysis and suggested to her that on the day her menstrual cycle began, she went outside but did not immerse herself in the cold water barrel; instead, she simply stood near it. He then brought her out of hypnosis and observed her until her next period. Miraculously, her menstrual cycle no longer accompanied the typical intense pain. This experiment led Janet to realize that he was touching upon some new, unexplored processes of our consciousness. To confirm his suspicions, he dared to conduct another experiment with the same patient, who had almost lost vision in her left eye at the age of six. Using a similar method of hypnoanalysis, Janet regressed the patient to the age of six and discovered that her symptoms began after an incident where her sick cousin, who had a skin condition, came to her home. Contrary to hygiene rules, her parents allowed her brother to sleep in the same bed with her, to her left. She described the intense negative feelings she experienced while lying in bed. Following this event, her vision in the left eye deteriorated almost to zero. In a hypnotic state, Janet suggested to the patient that her brother was completely healthy and that she was happy to see him. Over the next few months, he observed the restoration of her vision in the left eye.

In the future, Janet's findings were implemented by other hypnologists, who achieved similar successes at times, but often the restoration of vision through hypnosis was only temporary. We will delve further into this topic in subsequent chapters when discussing methods of vision therapy using hypnosis.

A notable student of the Nancy School and Hippolyte Bernheim was the French psychologist and pharmacist Émile Coué (1857–1926), who developed a system of psychotherapy based on self-hypnosis and autosuggestion.

Emile Coué's self-suggestion method involved the repeated recitation of healing phrases and affirmations aimed at improving or alleviating the patient's condition. An example of a phrase could be as follows: "Every day, in every way, I am getting better and better," "My health improves every day, regardless of what I do," "My intellect and physical strength constantly increase; I feel motivated to exercise, and I am full of energy." Coué tailored affirmations specifically for each patient or, if necessary, provided pre-prepared ones. The recommendation for the self-suggestion process was to regularly repeat the affirmation at least twenty times a day—in the morning, afternoon, and evening.

The duration could vary depending on the need and requirement, with the primary criterion being the patient's recovery. Therefore, the use of affirmations often continued for one to several weeks. Occasionally, Coué would recommend the continued use of affirmations as a preventive measure against illness. Naturally, affirmations could be utilized not only for the purpose of psychotherapy but also for personal growth.

Emile Coué (1857–1926)

Coué believed that the key to therapy lay in changing the patient's unconscious thinking. He emphasized that he himself is not a healer but merely teaches others to heal themselves. One of Coué's fundamental beliefs was that any person who suggests to themselves the phrase "I will succeed!" will inevitably achieve their desired outcome, despite criticism from the conscious mind and apparent external obstacles.

Another interesting belief held by Coué was that imagination triumphs over willpower, and whatever we envision as reality and affirm as reality through affirmation will eventually be realized.

Working as a pharmacist from 1882 to 1910, Coué made a remarkable discovery regarding the increased effectiveness of medication when presented to the patient as highly potent and reliable, compared to medications about which nothing was said. This finding anticipated the discovery of the placebo effect, which we will discuss in our book later on. This discovery marked the beginning of Coué's research in the fields of hypnosis and autosuggestion.

Coué also made the intriguing observation that a person cannot be hypnotized against their will, thus introducing a significant theoretical element to the theory of hypnosis. It is worth mentioning that other researchers of hypnosis were more inclined to talk about the individuals they successfully hypnotized than those with whom the phenomenon of hypnosis failed. Jean-Martin Charcot, Hippolyte Bernheim, and Auguste Liébeault, who predominantly worked with hysterical patients known for their exceptional hypnotic susceptibility, are often mentioned in the literature on hypnosis. However, the fact remains that individuals with different personality profiles sometimes encounter substantial difficulties in entering a trance state or are almost entirely incapable of doing so due to specific internal psychological processes. We will extensively discuss this topic in the chapter dedicated to personality profiling and its significance in the practice of hypnosis. This topic is highly significant but has been largely ignored and not discussed in the literature on hypnosis.

While offering tools for hypnotization, it is important to acknowledge that they may not work at all for individuals with certain profiles.

It is also worth mentioning that Emile Coué had a significant influence on Johann Heinrich Schultz (1884–1970), a German psychiatrist and psychotherapist who developed autogenic training. Schultz began practicing clinical hypnosis in 1909 and conducted various pathophysiological studies alongside it. Besides Emile Coué, he was greatly influenced by the works of Oscar Vogt and Sigmund Freud.

Johann Heinrich Schultz (1884–1970)

One of his major works was the book "Autogenic Training," published in 1932. It is noteworthy that the methods of autosuggestion and their application in psychotherapeutic practice were subsequently adopted worldwide.

One of his fundamental psychotherapeutic positions was the belief that therapy should take into account the "dynamic nature of the past" and the "current life situation of the individual patient."

The primary basic exercises in the autogenic training method involve the targeted creation of specific sensations in the body, such as warmth, cold, heaviness, and lightness, through self-suggestion, similar to the affirmations of Emile Coué. For example: "My hand is warm," "My hand is heavy," and so on. As the student developed the skill of inducing specific states through regular self-suggestion, more complex exercises were introduced.

One of the most intriguing personalities in the field of

practical hypnotic suggestion was Dave Elman (1900–1967), an American radio host, comedian, and singer. He taught numerous doctors the practice of hypnosis and wrote the book "Findings in Hypnosis" in 1964, later renamed "Hypnotherapy." D. Elman was famous for developing various forms of rapid hypnotic induction and adapting them for medical practice. It often took about three minutes to induce a hypnotic state using his methods.

It is also mentioned that the first heart surgery performed under hypnosis instead of anesthesia was conducted by one of D. Elman's students under his guidance. Further detailed information about this surgery is not available to us, but it is likely that the operation was carried out without general anesthesia, relying on local anesthesia, as this form of hypnotic work is now one of the most popular in clinics in France, Germany, England, and Italy.

Dave Elman (1900–1967)

Surgeries performed exclusively under local anesthesia using hypnosis on the heart are rare, as they require specific professional skills from the hypnotherapist and cannot be standardized. In less complex procedures, the use of hypnosis is very common nowadays because the hypnotization process is highly standardized and can be reproduced as a pattern even at lower levels of hypnotic practice competency. It should be noted that Dave Elman himself was neither a physician nor a psychologist; initially, his hypnotic techniques were aimed at creating a theatrical and demonstrative effect. Stage hypnosis is not considered a form of psychotherapy, as it emphasizes the creation of vivid hypnotic phenomena rather than therapeutic effects.

We should also mention the work of Swiss neurologist and psychiatrist Auguste Henri Forel in the field of hypnosis. Many of Forel's scientific research studies focused on topics such as the structure of the human central nervous system, hypnosis in psychotherapeutic practice, and other psychic phenomena. He worked as a professor of psychiatry in Zurich and was an honorary doctor of the University of Zurich. Some of his works were dedicated to combating alcohol addiction.

Auguste Henri Forel (1848–1931)

In this work, I would like to illustrate his use of hypnotherapy with a female patient suffering from severe menstrual pain, similar to the case of Pierre Janet. However, Forel employed a different approach compared to the intricate practice involving hypnotic regression and the implantation of false memories. He favored direct directive suggestion, wherein the symptom was alleviated through the direct suggestion of the desired state. According to the patient's description, her menstruation typically lasted over a week and was accompanied by intense pain. Over the course of several weeks, Forel conducted a series of hypnosis sessions with her, repeatedly suggesting that her menstruation would be reduced to three days, become moderate in intensity, and be nearly painless. As he later reported, the patient's subsequent menstrual cycles corresponded to the suggestions he had given her.

It is worth noting that when examining the works of early hypnotherapists, one can find numerous examples of successful practices in both hypnosis and symptom elimination, with very few descriptions of unsuccessful attempts. It is reasonable to assume that some challenges in practice were simply left undocumented. While hypnosis can yield astonishing results in the short term, it frequently leads to the regression of "rapid healing," with the reemergence of old symptoms. Understanding such regression phenomena often lies in the concept of the positive intention underlying the symptom.

To further illustrate this point, allow me to share a case from my own practice involving a 60-year-old male patient, a high-ranking military officer, who was grappling with severe alcoholism. This patient demonstrated a high level of hypnotizability, readily entering into a deep hypnotic state. The induction of a simple trance state alone had a positive therapeutic effect, resulting in a significant reduction in his alcohol consumption over several months of weekly hypnotherapy sessions. It is important to note that the patient, while conscious, was resistant to the complete elimination of his addiction, asserting his strong willpower and attributing hypnosis as a tool only for the weak-minded. Consequently, we opted for a strategy that avoided direct interventions aimed at countering the addiction, such as suggestions like "you do not want to drink alcohol" or "alcohol repulses you."

During the hypnosis sessions, we focused on motivational interventions, emphasizing the healing of his mind and body. We provided suggestions such as "your body and mind are undergoing a process of healing," "you no longer have the desire to harm your body," and "your consciousness is becoming more integrated and healthy." After several successful hypnotherapy sessions, we cautiously attempted to suggest to the patient, while he was in a deep hypnotic trance, the phrase "vodka is poison to you." To our surprise, he immediately emerged from the trance and expressed a strong desire to terminate the session. It became evident that the patient, perhaps unconsciously, was fiercely protecting his addiction.

In a subsequent hypnosis session, we explored the patient's memories of early breastfeeding by his mother, uncovering a significant psychological factor underlying his alcohol dependency. It is worth digressing and commenting that some alcoholics unconsciously associate alcohol with the comforting experience of maternal milk, attempting to recreate the sense of well-being from their childhood. Alcohol, like maternal milk, triggers the release of neurotransmitters such as GABA, oxytocin, and dopamine in the brain, which can serve as an "adult" substitute for the emotional nourishment they seek. Attempting to directly eliminate alcohol dependence without providing alternative psychological resources deprives the individual of the opportunity for psychological balance. Without appropriate substitutes, the symptom is likely to resurface.

Let's take a simple example from our practice with a 60-year-old male patient, a professional general, who suffered from severe alcoholism. The man was capable of consuming up to three bottles of vodka per night, coming home after work. He was referred for treatment by his family members. During the hypnotic work, he exhibited a high level of hypnotizability and easily entered a hypnotic state. Simple immersion in a hypnotic trance had a healing effect. Over the course of several months, conducting weekly hypnotherapy sessions, we observed a significant reduction in the amount of alcohol the patient consumed.

It is worth noting that in his conscious state, he did not want to completely rid himself of his addiction, justifying it by claiming that he was a strong-willed individual and capable of overcoming the dependency on his own. He believed that only weak-willed people resorted to "coding" through hypnosis. Due to this, we chose a strategy of avoiding direct interventions that curbed the addiction, such as suggesting statements like "you don't want to drink alcohol," "alcohol disgusts you," "you feel nauseous at the smell of alcohol," and so on. For a while, we provided motivational interventions during the hypnotic state, such as "your body and mind are healing," "you have no desire to harm your body," "your consciousness becomes more whole and healthy."

When several successful hypnotherapy sessions were established, we attempted to implant the phrase "vodka is poison to you" while the patient was in a deep hypnotic trance. We witnessed the instant emergence of the patient from the trance and his desire to leave. It was evident that the patient, seemingly unconsciously, was "protecting his addiction." In one of the subsequent hypnotherapy sessions, we discovered the patient's memories of early breastfeeding, a process underlying the need to consume alcohol. At this point, it is worth making a brief digression and commenting that, indeed, some alcoholics unconsciously project the qualities of maternal milk onto alcohol, attempting to recreate the sense of well-being experienced during infancy. Alcohol, like maternal milk, can stimulate the production of neurotransmitters such as GABA, oxytocin, and dopamine in the brain, easily becoming an "adult" substitute for the latter in emotionally challenging situations for an individual.

Attempting to directly eliminate a person's alcohol dependency merely deprives them of alternative psychological balancing, and if no substitutes are provided, the symptom will resurface or manifest in another, sometimes more destructive, form. The same applied to our patient when we asked him how it happened that he frequently consumed alcohol. He mentioned that his life consisted of a constant circulation between work-related stress and conflicts in the domestic sphere. Alcohol dependency had become the only means of relaxation for an extended period. In this case, we observe the conscious inclination to protect one's addiction. In numerous other similar patients, we discover similar, often unconscious processes that cannot be corrected without additional verbal psychotherapy. In this regard, hypnosis appears as a tool that can facilitate change only when the patient's unconscious is ready to accept it. If the hypnotic suggestion does not resonate with the hidden beliefs and values of the patient, we often witness a regression to the previous symptom after a certain period of time. Although, based on our observations, there are many hypnosis specialists claiming to be able to cure alcoholism without analytical correction, we question such beliefs, considering the impossibility of directly resolving the underlying situation that led to the dependent behavior. In the practical part of the book, we will delve deeper into the specifics of hypnotic psychotherapeutic work and the factors contributing to the emergence of addictive behavior.

Milton Erickson (1901–1988)

One of the most renowned psychiatrists and hypnotherapists of the 20th century was the American physician Milton Erickson (1901–1988), the creator of the non-directive form of hypnosis and an entire direction of psychotherapy named after him.

A particularly interesting aspect of his biography was his childhood illness, poliomyelitis. At that time, this disease had no known cure, and its presence often implied a fatal outcome. He overheard a doctor commenting to his mother that he would not survive until the next day. However, contrary to the doctor's expectations, he continued to live, paralyzed and only capable of thinking and moving his eyes. His mother placed his bed in the kitchen of their home so she could attend to her duties while keeping an eye on her son. Milton, lying in bed, exerted his willpower and imagination to suggest to himself that he could move his fingers. After some time, he succeeded. Then he managed to convince himself that he could move all his limbs and eventually his entire body. Against all odds, he gradually recovered, although he remained in considerable pain. Milton faced several physical challenges. In addition to poliomyelitis, which appeared when he was 17, he suffered from color blindness and difficulty distinguishing sounds by pitch. As Milton grew up and entered medical school, where he later specialized in psychiatry, one of his professors told him that he would be an excellent psychiatrist. Milton inquired about the reason for such a statement, and the professor replied that Milton was small, sickly, and unattractive. Therefore, he would not arouse a desire to compete among men, and women would feel sympathy for him, making them more likely to collaborate with him. Despite the absurdity of this assumption, his mentor turned out to be right in many respects. It is worth adding that Milton's fame and success did not come early in his life.

Milton Erickson first encountered clinical hypnosis while serving as a medical intern and observing the work of the American psychologist and hypnotherapist Clark Hull. It is difficult to assess the influence of C. Hull on Milton Erickson's work since Milton never mentioned him in his writings or acknowledged using his methods. Perhaps at the beginning of his professional journey, Milton did utilize directive suggestion methods borrowed from C. Hull. However, most of what we know about Milton Erickson's hypnotherapy is that he developed the majority of his methods independently within the context of his psychotherapeutic practice.

A very interesting experiment was conducted by M. Erickson in 1936, where he observed how a person creates associations with a stimulus word that directly describes their problem. For example, one of his patients associated the word "stomach" with words like pain, worry, baby, fear, surgery, illness, and forgotten. These associations reflected information about her

40

unwanted pregnancy, which she had forgotten.

After his research, M. Erickson hypothesized that it is possible to interact with the patient's unconscious from a different "riverbank" by giving them hinting words related to a specific process or command. Thus, through indirect suggestion rather than direct and directive means, the patient's resistance is bypassed. This study laid the foundation for his exploration and development of his own method of hypnotherapy, which significantly differed from the methods previously known in psychotherapy. His approach prioritized indirect suggestions and metaphors. M. Erickson referred to his technique as "hypnotic trance" rather than "hypnosis," verbally distinguishing his method of hypnotic suggestion, which went beyond ordinary suggestion. However, it would be incorrect to say that M. Erickson exclusively used nondirective methods. Rather, he elegantly combined his working styles based on their appropriateness. M. Erickson believed that the state of hypnotic trance is a natural tool of consciousness necessary for processing internal experience. The act of entering a hypnotic state itself can have a healing effect. Despite this, he developed numerous procedures that could be performed in a trance state to accelerate the healing process.

Erickson specialized in creating various hypnotic phenomena that could be utilized either to demonstrate trance phenomenology or to act as triggers for entering a trance state and directing the healing process. His favorite trance phenomena included catalepsy of the hand, which allowed flexibility in positioning the hand and maintaining that position for a period of time without the patient's conscious effort, and levitation of the hand, an unconscious movement of the hand in the air characterized by autonomous lifting and a certain duration

41

of movement. M. Erickson conducted many experiments in creating anesthesia and analgesia phenomena, both on himself due to his own illness and on his patients, especially those suffering from cancer. While he could not cure cancer through hypnosis, he could alleviate some of the patients' suffering. He also actively practiced the creation of other trance phenomena, such as positive and negative visual hallucinations, hypnotic hypermnesia and amnesia, nonverbal analog body signals, and so on. We will discuss them in more detail in the section of the book dedicated to the phenomenology of hypnotic trance.

Erickson became famous only in the last 20 years of his professional career. He never sought fame but diligently worked with patients, often doing remarkable things that genuinely helped them. In the modern world, M. Erickson is primarily known for his methods of hypnotic induction, but hypnosis was just one of the many tools he used in psychotherapy. He didn't use hypnosis with many of his patients, instead employing direct and behavioral metaphors to correct their behavior. It is worth providing examples of some of these techniques, which are not direct hypnosis but reflect the essence of his therapeutic work.

Once upon a time, a man came to M. Erickson and complained that he was an alcoholic and couldn't quit drinking. He mentioned that many members of his family were heavy drinkers, as were his colleagues at work. He constantly found himself in contexts where alcohol was present, which led to him being drawn back into the "alcohol pit" even when he tried to abstain. M. Erickson pondered for a while and then said he could help him, but first, the man had to promise to carry out an assignment despite its outward strangeness and peculiarity. The man agreed immediately. M. Erickson instructed him to go to the city's botanical garden and find the section dedicated to cacti. He was to walk through that section, look at the cacti, examine these plants closely, and contemplate how they could survive for up to two years without water. He was to walk, observe, and think, think, think... The patient agreed to fulfill M. Erickson's directive and left his office. After that, M. Erickson didn't hear from him for six years.

Six years later, a young woman knocked on M. Erickson's office door and asked where she could find Dr. M. Erickson. He asked her why she wanted to see him, and she replied that she had long wanted to meet the doctor who had advised an alcoholic patient to go to the botanical garden, look at the cacti, and then quit drinking.

In this case, we observe that M. Erickson created a behavioral metaphor for the patient that was embedded with images and profound meanings that were most likely not consciously understood by the patient. However, his unconscious mind found interpretations for them and manifested the effect at the level of neurophysiological reactions. The alcoholic himself served as an analogy to the cactus, and alcohol served as an analogy to water. Two years without water symbolized the ability to exert willpower to overcome addiction. This work by M. Erickson, if we think about it, carries even more meaning than we can imagine. Initially, we discover the rule that metaphors encode our subconscious and enable us to do one thing and not do another. M. Erickson believed that what the patient did not consciously grasp influenced him much more than conscious realizations. He substantiated his theory through his practice and examples, although he also believed that psychotherapy could not afford the luxury of having rigid theoretical frameworks regarding personality theory and psychotherapeutic methods.

Many psychotherapists believe that M. Erickson contributed as much to the practice of psychotherapy as Sigmund Freud contributed to its theory. In many ways, this statement holds true. We can learn a lot about patients from both Freud's and Erickson's psychotherapeutic sources. With Freud, we do not find descriptions of patients' recovery but mostly theorizing and constructing models of personality. M. Erickson rarely engaged in theoretical discussions. However, his work often resulted in the actual healing of the patient.

Another question that arises after considering the case of working with an alcoholic is whether the metaphor, whose meaning is not consciously grasped, can help a person exert willpower. In that case, what is primary?

It turns out that the unconscious metaphorical experience of a person completely determines their ability to exercise will, life motivation, behavioral reactions, and the meanings we attribute to the world. Does freedom of choice exist in such a scenario, or does the overwhelming majority of a person's reactions relate to the reproduction of unconscious metaphorical experience? On one hand, the answer may seem philosophical, but on the other hand, it constructs an entirely new map for describing the hierarchy of neurophysiological processes in the human brain. Metaphors, as complete programs living in a person's consciousness, acting as algorithms for both psychological and neurophysiological processes, seem capable of encoding processes of volition and many other behavioral processes in humans.

As another interesting example of M. Erickson's non-hypnotic work, which vividly illustrates our concept of the primacy of unconscious metaphorical experience in relation to the process of volition, let's consider his work with a high jumper who needed to learn how to jump half a meter farther than he believed he was capable of. M. Erickson discovered that the athlete had developed a belief in his inability to overcome this barrier during training and competitions. Whenever the athlete thought about the need to jump half a meter farther than his best performance to win a competition, he would become discouraged and lose motivation, and naturally, his athletic performance would not improve.

Erickson attempted to shake his limiting beliefs about his abilities in the following way. The first question he would ask him was, "Do you think you can jump one centimeter farther than your record? Can you overcome this barrier?" The athlete confidently replied that he saw nothing impossible about it. M. Erickson then assigned him the task of trying to add that one centimeter to his record over the next week. And miraculously, after a week of training, the athlete achieved a new record with an additional centimeter. M. Erickson then asked him to try adding one or two centimeters to his new record every week. The athlete successfully completed the tasks, and in six months, he finally jumped half a meter farther than his initial limit. In this situation, we observe how M. Erickson worked on reshaping the patient's belief about his inability to overcome the barrier, demonstrating that it resided more in the individual's mind and was not directly linked to his true abilities. Here we can recall the old psychotherapeutic metaphor: "How do you eat an elephant? One bite at a time." It is an elegant alternative approach to working with the patient's consciousness, not relying on literal hypnotic suggestion but nonetheless reprogramming the patient's mind as effectively, and possibly even better, than direct directive suggestion that a clinical directive hypnotist might employ. These cases primarily serve as examples of a psychotherapist's ability to work with the patient's resistance, a process that often poses a significant stumbling block for many psychotherapists.

In our experience, we have witnessed hypnotic triumphs and "fails" by highly successful hypnotherapists. If the structure of resistance is not understood and acknowledged by the hypnotherapist and the patient's personality profile is not taken into account, the process of hypnotherapy becomes akin to playing "Russian roulette," with the thought, "What if it backfires?" After all, clear and fixed hypnotic methods, both directive and non-directive, can have varying effects on patients' consciousness. Here are a few vivid examples from our practice.

One patient who underwent psychotherapy with us requested to be hypnotized in order to assess her hypnotizability. In the hypnotic work with her, we initially adopted the style of a gentle, non-directive Ericksonian approach, where the process of hypnotization is carried out with a slow, gentle, and calm voice. After ten minutes of work, we observed that such delivery of suggestions did not work on the patient; she constantly experienced anxious reactions that disrupted her hypnotic state. Intrigued by her resistance, we engaged in a conversation to understand what was happening in her consciousness when anxiety arose. It turned out that the patient, who had conflicting relationships with her mother, had an interesting association related to her mother's voice. Her mother always used a soft and calm voice to tell her what to do and what not to do. This always frustrated her, and in her mind, this type of voice became associated with her mother's attempts to give her advice or commands that were unpleasant

46

to her.

This is an example of how even the most comfortable and non-intrusive form of hypnotic work can encounter "hidden reefs" of resistance associated with the patient's personal experience.

Another example comes from a seminar on Ericksonian hypnotic work that we conducted. During the seminar, one of our hypnotherapist colleagues participated in a demonstration of trance induction for the group of participants. When we asked him for feedback on the effectiveness of the hypnotic induction, we encountered a situation where certain hypnotic phrases from the non-directive Ericksonian hypnosis, which we used abundantly, unconsciously irritated our colleague. He commented that he was quite familiar with the examples of hypnotic interventions used in the Ericksonian style, and when he heard them being applied to him, he began to resist the hypnotic induction, explaining that he felt manipulated. In a subsequent personal conversation with him, we discovered that throughout his life, he had been subjected to various manipulations from his mother, manipulations that he was well aware of. There were many emotions involved, and he needed to redirect them somewhere. Verbal, non-directive Ericksonian interventions became the victim. According to his personal comments, when direct imperative hypnosis was applied to him, where the suggestion was always evident on the surface, it symbolized sincerity and a lack of desire to manipulate him. In this case, he entered the hypnotic trance easily and effortlessly.

Erickson often utilized behavioral metaphors to alter patients perceptions. It is important to emphasize that he achieved success not only with neurotic patients but also with severely psychotic individuals. One such case involved a thirteen-year-old girl who was admitted to the clinic due to intense, aggressive outbursts, making it nearly impossible for the medical staff to interact with her. She would lunge at doctors and nurses, attempting to bite them and pull their hair. When left alone in her room, she would tear apart the bedding and break furniture.

Erickson aimed to develop a therapeutic approach and establish a connection with her based on three fundamental principles that guided both his hypnotic and behavioral therapy. These principles were: joining the patient's behavior, leading them through its expression, and therapeutic utilization.

Erickson coordinated with the clinic director to shut off the hot water supply to the radiator in the girl's room and enlisted the help of a specific nurse to assist him in a particular form of behavioral therapy for the patient. He then entered the girl's room and initiated a conversation with her. Sitting on the bed, she glared at him with hostility, ready to attack. Sensing her readiness to express aggression, Erickson grabbed the bed sheets and tore them apart in front of her with ferocious intensity. She was taken aback by this display. He then seized a pillow, ripped it open, and scattered feathers throughout the room. The girl was astounded by what she witnessed. She had never seen herself from an external perspective while engaging in similar destructive behavior. Seizing the opportunity, Erickson invited her to participate in the "destruction" of the bedding. After a while, the girl joined him in this destructive tandem. Thirty minutes later, they celebrated their accomplishment as the bedding was completely destroyed. Erickson then suggested dismantling the radiator from the wall, and after another half hour of struggling, they successfully achieved this as well. By that point, the girl saw Erickson as a close friend. Urging her to take a walk in the corridor, Erickson hurried to the door, and she eagerly followed him. Waiting outside the door was the "prepared" nurse, who had willingly agreed to participate in this eccentric form of psychotherapy. Erickson rushed toward her, grabbing her by the sleeves of her coat and abruptly tearing them off. The patient observed her therapist's destructive behavior without actively participating, feeling a mild sense of fear. After a brief moment of confusion, she asked him, "Dr. Erickson, are you sure it's okay to do this?"

Numerous stories like this can be found in Milton Erickson's books, where he successfully aligned himself with the behavior of even the most irrational patients, bringing them back to an appropriate state of mind. Erickson recognized in his psychotherapeutic practice that patients truly started to listen and hear him only when he shared their reality, no matter how outrageous it may have been. To be understood, one must learn to speak the language of the other person. If one desires others to follow, they must first lead by following someone else. If one wants someone to share their cousin's story, they should share their own story first. A similar analogy was applied during trance interactions with patients: "If you want to induce someone into trance, first enter into trance yourself." These beliefs significantly differentiated Erickson's therapy and hypnosis methods from those of other therapists, who rarely employed such principles.

It is important to note that in Ericksonian hypnosis, rapport primarily focuses on aligning with the patient, contrasting with classical directive hypnosis, where the concepts of rapport and trust could be interpreted differently. It is worth mentioning that Anton Mesmer initially regarded rapport as the process of transmitting magnetic fluid from the hypnotist to the patient through physical contact. According to Erickson, rapport primarily involves sharing the patient's reality. It represents an entirely different level of working with resistance and the therapeutic process.

The therapeutic approach of M. Erickson's philosophy shares similarities with the philosophy of the ancient Chinese philosopher Lao Tzu. However, it is doubtful that Lao Tzu's works directly influenced M. Erickson's professional development. In this case, an appropriate aphorism by Lao Tzu would be as follows:

"Many mountain rivers flow into the deep sea. The reason is that the seas are lower than the mountains. Therefore, they can govern all the streams. Similarly, a wise person, desiring to be above others, becomes lower than them. Wanting to be in front, they position themselves behind. Thus, although their place is above others, they do not feel burdened by it. Although their place is in front, others do not perceive it as unfair."

In addition to the use of the key concepts of joining, leading, and utilization, M. Erickson was an advocate of the antipsychiatric philosophy in psychotherapeutic practice. This philosophy takes a softer approach to the understanding of pathological behavior and places the primary goal of therapy not in conforming the patient to traditional standards of health, but in their social adaptation within society. It matters little whether a person thinks they are Napoleon or sees things that aren't there; what is important is their ability to be socially adapted and derive pleasure from life.

An example of M. Erickson's antipsychiatric psychotherapeutic work is as follows: On one occasion, M. Erickson had the opportunity to work with a patient who believed he was Jesus

Christ. M. Erickson asked him, "Are you Jesus?" The patient replied, "Yes, of course!" M. Erickson then said, "Listen, I have a job for you. They're building an extension next to the clinic, and they need a carpenter. Can you help?" What do you think Jesus replied to? Of course, he said "Yes."

"But I will ask one thing of you: please do not tell people that you are Jesus. It will frighten them, as they are not yet ready to comprehend exactly who is before them. Can you do this for them?" posed another question by M. Erickson. The patient agreed joyfully. For six months, he worked as a carpenter, concealing his "true" identity. During this time, the patient behaved normally, and his claims of involvement in events from the New Testament were no longer heard from him.

Psychiatrists decided to form a commission to interview the patient and inquire about how his perception of the world had changed in order to determine whether to release him from the clinic or keep him further. M. Erickson persuaded the patient not to disclose his "true" name to the doctors and instead use only the name from his passport. It was for their own good, of course, as this way he would be able to leave the clinic and spread goodness in the world. And, of course, if they were to release him, he was not to tell others but simply act as Jesus. To do good and help others. The patient went through the commission, left the clinic, moved to another city, and eventually established a community to aid and support those in need, becoming highly successful and sought-after in this field. Every year, on Christmas, he would write a lengthy greeting card to Milton H. Erickson, expressing gratitude for his assistance. At the bottom of the letter, he would sign his name as it appeared on his passport but would always add the initials "J.C" (Jesus Christ) in lowercase.

We won't claim that such a therapeutic approach could be effective in many other cases of schizophrenic personality disorder. Each case of illness can be highly individual and require an individualized approach to treating the symptoms. The depth of the psychiatric symptom and the patient's intellectual level will naturally have a significant influence. However, M. Erickson's work demonstrated at times that even a patient who initially seemed resistant to therapy could, with proper assistance, find their path to healing.

Naturally, M. Erickson effectively applied the technique of joining the patient's state during direct hypnotization. Through this method, he was occasionally able to hypnotize patients who exhibited strong resistance, even those who consciously resisted. Contrary to Emil Coué's belief that if a patient intentionally resists, it would likely be impossible to induce a hypnotic state. However, M. Erickson was truly a master of hypnotic tricks. Here's an example of one of the most amusing ones. One day, a man entered M. Erickson's office and asked him to try to hypnotize him. He was curious whether M. Erickson could succeed. Accepting the challenge, M. Erickson fully understood that the man would consciously resist. He attempted to hypnotize him using several standard methods that were typical for him, and he became convinced that the man was a tough nut to crack and the usual hypnotization methods would not work. Then he told the man that he would step out for a couple of minutes, left the office, and went to the reception area where his secretary was sitting. He quickly induced her into a deep trance state and suggested that she go into his office, sit across from the man, and gaze intently into his eyes until he entered a state of deep hypnotic trance. She left. M. Erickson refrained from entering his office for a while and drank tea. When he finally entered, he saw two people sitting on chairs in a very deep trance state.

Resistance to trance induction is always directed towards something. It could be towards the person themselves—their gender, hair color, social hierarchy, body position, and so on.

In this case, M. Erickson simply assumed that all the resistance was directed towards him personally. The patient came to him specifically to demonstrate their ability to resist him, not the young female secretary who unexpectedly became his hypnotist.

We could provide numerous examples of such fixed resistance. Let us share an interesting one from our experience.

A few years ago, we conducted a hypnotic laboratory where we experimented with the ability to memorize large amounts of information in a hypnotic state. We invited a large number of our students to participate in the experiment. Some of the students who had previously participated in the experiment had experienced hypnotic states, while others came to try trance for the first time.

When we worked with a novice female student, we found that the first few minutes of hypnotic speech had no effect on her state at all. She continued to sit, look at us, and blink, showing no signs of a hypnotic trance. We continued our hypnotic work, fully confident in our abilities.

The next five minutes showed that our efforts still had no desired effect. The student clearly resisted trance induction strongly. We continued the hypnotic speech as if she were already in a trance, despite her reactions. None of the tricks we tried worked on her. This situation persisted even after fifteen minutes.

The audience became nervous, but we continued our work as if there were no resistance. Finally, as our last attempt at hypnotic work, we set a verbal frame, saying that we would count from ten to one, and when we reached one, the girl would exit the trance state (even though she was still awake). When we uttered the word "one," her eyes closed and her head slightly tilted forward. She entered a hypnotic trance.

We continued to work with her for another fifteen minutes, accomplishing our research goal. This is an example of para-doxical induction. The girl's resistance persisted until the hypnotic frame was established. As soon as she heard that she could exit the trance, it signaled her to stop resisting hypnotic induction.

While such examples are not common in practice, they vividly illustrate M. Erickson's concepts for working with patient resistance.

Ericksonian hypnotic style is focused on finding an adequate method of hypnotic induction. If one approach doesn't work, another one might. The key is to understand what the client's resistance is directed towards and to select an appropriate method of hypnotic work. However, it is worth admitting that even for M. Erickson himself, the search for a method sometimes took more than a day.

When we talk about the key techniques of rapport-building with the patient during hypnosis in the works of M. Erickson, it is worth mentioning the practices he developed for matching the patient's postures, movements, and breathing. These techniques became particularly popular thanks to the work of M. Erickson's students, R. Bandler and J. Grinder, who later created Neuro-Linguistic Programming (NLP) and made these techniques a fundamental tool in their methodology.

If we covertly mimic the patient's movements and postures for an extended period, a sense of identity between themselves and us may begin to arise in their consciousness. What is in a similar rhythm to me—either I myself or someone close to me whom I can trust. Any shared rhythms inspire trust, and the more there are, the greater the trust grows. Matching the depth and rhythm of breathing has a similar effect. A vivid example that illustrates matching body posture and breathing is a case of psychotherapeutic work by one of Milton Erickson's students, John Grinder, who once tried to use these techniques to bring a catatonic schizophrenic out of a stupor in a psychiatric clinic.

During catatonia, a schizophrenic can sit in one place for many hours without reacting to the world, words, or actions of others. In the overwhelming majority of cases, any attempts to rouse them have no effect. If you place them in a different posture, they will maintain it without exiting the stuporous state. John Grinder decided to match the patient's posture and breathing—the only criteria that could be mirrored in his behavior. For forty minutes, he simply sat next to the schizophrenic, adopting his posture and breathing in rhythm with him. Then he lightly tapped him on the shoulder and said, "Give me a cigarette." The schizophrenic came out of the stupor, turned towards him, and replied that he didn't smoke. Prior to this, any direct attempts by doctors to bring him out of the stuporous state had not yielded any constructive results. It is worth commenting a bit on this case, as we believe that John Grinder took some risks, as not all catatonic schizophrenics behave peacefully when they come out of the catatonic stupor. There is always a high probability of aggressive actions towards others when their catatonia is interrupted. However, this does not imply the ineffectiveness of the "awakening" method for patients. It rather emphasizes the importance of precautionary methods that need to be observed when reproducing such practices with severely psychotic patients.

2

Psychopathological Profile of Hypnotizable Individuals

Since the times of Anton Mesmer, James Braid, Jean-Martin Charcot, Hippolyte Bernheim, and Ambroise-Auguste Liebeault, doctors have noticed that some patients exhibit extremely high hypnotizability, entering a state of deep hypnotic trance either instantly or within a few minutes. With other patients, it takes some effort to induce a hypnotic trance, and there have always been individuals who show such strong unconscious resistance that the best methods, which worked on others, fail when attempting to hypnotize them. Initially, practitioners of hypnosis were perplexed by the reasons behind these vastly different effects.

The initial models of hypnotizability and non-hypnotizability were limited to elementary attempts at classifying individuals as either neurologically predisposed or not predisposed to the process of hypnosis. In contemporary literature, remnants of such notions can still be found, where readers are presented with "clinical" data stating, for example, that 15% of people are highly hypnotizable, 70% are moderately hypnotizable, and the remaining 15% are weakly hypnotizable or non-hypnotizable altogether. While these figures may vary in different sources, you will generally find similar data. However, such data is absurd considering that these studies did not take into account a multitude of factors that could be crucial in the creation of such clinical data.

What are these factors? For example, what was the composition of the individuals involved in these studies? Were they male or female? Were they physically healthy or ill? Similarly, were they mentally healthy or not? If some of them were ill, what were their illnesses, and to what extent did they affect them? What were their cultural and national backgrounds? What social class did they belong to? What were their ages? Were they religious or atheists? What kind of upbringing did they have in their childhood, and what was their relationship with parental figures in the family? Did they experience any aggressive physical or sexual abuse during their lifetime?

Furthermore, a key omission in compiling such statistics was the question of who exactly hypnotized the people included in the aforementioned statistics. Was it one specialist? Two? Ten? What was the level of their competence? What methods did they use during hypnosis? Was there a single method employed for everyone, or did it vary? Did some of them utilize different styles of hypnotic work? What were the gender and age of the hypnotists themselves? We assert that depending on these factors, the level of hypnotizability would vary significantly. As you can understand, creating a comprehensive statistical database that could yield meaningful correlations among these criteria is very challenging, if not impossible.

Our research data indicates that understanding the key characteristics of psychoanalytic, psychopathological, cultural-ethnic, and socio-cultural profiles can provide highly accurate predictions regarding the majority of hypnotizability and non-hypnotizability criteria in individuals. In this book, we aim to present a comprehensive integrative model of conceptualizations concerning the key predisposing factors for entering the hypnotic trance.

Let's begin with an elementary discussion of the afore-mentioned criteria and initially focus on the clinical data obtained by the earliest researchers in the field of hypnosis in clinical practice. Physicians observed that women are much more susceptible to hypnotic suggestion than men, with deeper and more intense trance states. Unfortunately, we did not find logical explanations for this phenomenon in the literature. To evaluate this phenomenon, it is necessary to turn to contemporary findings in the field of neurophysiology and pay attention to the connection between the hypnotic state and the activities of various brain regions. In the 1940s, a model of the brain emerged in neurophysiology that divided our brain into three main sectors:

1. **Archicortex**
2. **Limbic system**
3. **Neocortex (**or simply the cortex)

This model was named the triune brain model. The archicorti-cal region is predominantly associated with our instinctive activities, processing basic elementary movements and actions, and actualizing needs for food, water, sleep, and sexual relationships. This brain region was also referred to as the "reptilian brain" since scientists believe it originated in reptiles and then passed on to primates and eventually to humans through evolution. The activity of this brain region is inherited through the evolutionary process. Reptiles experience almost no emotions and are primarily oriented towards instinctual behavior (previously we would have said they experience no emotions at all, but in the context of modern research, we can say they do not experience them as higher animals and humans do, although some signs of emotional processes can still be traced at the neurochemical level in reptiles). Emotional activity emerges in animals with the development of a new brain region, the limbic system, which gives rise to various emotional processes. Animals are capable of experiencing anger, fear, joy, etc., which naturally influences their activities and is not solely based on the instinctual processes of the archicortex. At the level of activity in the limbic system and the beginnings of the neocortex, animals are already capable of performing certain types of activities that can be evaluated as forms of thinking. Modern ethology suggests that the intelligence of higher primates is sometimes comparable to that of 4-6-year-old children. These animals are capable of receiving feedback from the external world and performing activities not typical of their species in order to solve a given task. Although we could provide numerous examples of intellectual activities in animals and birds, we will refrain from delving into this topic as it would deviate from the essence of our research. Let us focus on the fact that the emergence of the neocortex, that is, the full development of the cerebral hemispheres, enables humans to enhance the intellectual capabilities inherent in animals and make verbal thinking possible.

Research on the neurophysiology of hypnotic states and other altered states of consciousness shows that when a person is able to immerse themselves in a state of hypnotic trance, the activity of the cerebral cortex of the brain's hemispheres dampens to some extent, while greater activity is observed in the subcortex. The less active the cerebral cortex, the deeper and more uncontrollable the trance state we can achieve. The higher its activity, the more superficial and controllable the trance becomes.

This information allows for numerous conclusions to be drawn. For example, one might assume that the more verbal and cognitive activity a person exhibits, the less susceptible they are to hypnosis. However, this is not entirely true. The verbal and cognitive domains and their level of development do not directly determine the possible depth of hypnotic induction.

But if we consider individuals whose line of work or life experiences require them to focus their thinking around the theme of self-preservation, we will find that attempting to hypnotize such individuals presents certain challenges. The activity of the cerebral cortex in these individuals has become part of their survival strategy, and ceasing to think about danger or relinquishing conscious control over the situation is synonymous with death or something similar. This process is almost always evident in people suffering from paranoid personality disorder. Paranoid individuals are among the worst subjects for hypnosis.

In contrast, schizoid personalities, who also predominantly live in their "heads" and exhibit heightened activity in the cerebral cortex, can display very deep trance states with properly constructed hypnotic suggestions, temporarily releasing the activity of the cerebral cortex.

Let's return to the topic of men and women and provide data from a highly specific neurophysiological study in the field of sexology. Scientists became interested in understanding what happens in the human brain when experiencing an orgasm and how these processes differ between men and women. We will not delve into the specifics of this study, but we will comment on the fact that brain activity during orgasm does indeed differ between men and women.

What is the main difference? During orgasm, the cerebral cortex in the vast majority of cases is only partially deactivated in men. On the contrary, in women, the cortex's activity is more often completely deactivated during orgasm, allowing them to experience more sensations (particularly pleasure) from sex and, naturally, be less aware of them due to the absence of control.

A philosophical question arises: what is better or worse? To experience more pleasure but not be fully aware of what one is experiencing, or to experience less pleasure but be conscious of what is happening.

There was a Greek legend about whether men or women derive more pleasure from sex. Once, a Greek hero was walking through the forest when he came across two mating snakes. He threw a stick at them, interrupting their sexual act. The gods witnessed his act and punished him by transforming him into a woman for nine years (apparently, becoming a woman was considered a punishment in ancient Greece). Our hero lived as a woman for nine years and then transformed back into a man.

Afterward, he was asked, "Having been both a man and a woman and having engaged in lovemaking in these roles, tell us, who derives more pleasure from sex?" He replied, "A woman derives nine times more pleasure." The legend might have seemed like a beautiful story if it weren't for modern neurophysiological studies, which partly seem to confirm its veracity.

Naturally, if we observe similar neurophysiological effects in the majority of women, it indicates a genetic factor predisposing them to this. We can make an assumption as to why such a division occurs. In the context of evolution, men, being hunters, warriors, and protectors, often died if they lost control of their primary sphere of activity. Even during lovemaking, ancient men had to remain vigilant to ensure their own safety and the safety of their wives. More vigilant men survived more often than inattentive ones. Thus, through natural selection, the careless were eliminated. Women, on the other hand, did not have the need to be overly vigilant since they relied on men beside them to fulfill this function.

Based on the given information, we can assert that the behavior of the brain during orgasm, specifically whether self-control is inhibited during sex, provides us with a comprehensive understanding of an individual's capacity to immerse themselves in a hypnotic trance or other altered states of consciousness and the depth they can reach.

In our practice, while working with a significant number of men, we have made intriguing findings when encountering highly hypnotizable individuals. Almost all of them had some involvement with cult religious organizations at some point in their lives. These men were capable of delving into the deepest levels of hypnotic trance, performing various phenomena, and being unaware of what was happening to them. On the one hand, they were intellectually developed, indicating a high level of development in the cerebral cortex of the brain's hemispheres. On the other hand, it appears that their cerebral cortex could be deactivated, similar to women with hysterical disorders. We hypothesized that trance-inducing rituals in religions train the human brain to engage

63

in trance-like processes. Whether it involves chanting, mantra recitation, prayers, and so on, the human mind is capable of learning to disable self-control (meta-self-control). When such individuals participate in a hypnotic session, even if it is their first experience of being hypnotized, their brains are already accustomed to this form of activity. In our opinion, in ancient communities, particularly shamans, individuals who practiced trance rituals learned to deeply deactivate the activity of the cerebral cortex, enabling them to access numinous revelations during trance states, which subsequently formed the foundation of religious beliefs. By the way, some contemporary psychiatrists perceive the activities of shamans as manifestations of hysteria and epilepsy, disorders that often provide fertile ground for hypnotic suggestion and the reproduction of various hypnotic phenomena. This serves as an example of the differentiation between male and female profiles.

It is worth noting that the resistance of some men to the process of hypnotization is at times linked to particular beliefs about the correlation between susceptibility to hypnosis and personal strength. This rigidity can be especially noticeable in men with wounded masculine egos, where feelings of inadequacy are profound. If a man is hypnotized by another man, it can become another confirmation of his perceived inadequacy. However, this rule is not absolute, and variations and nuances can be observed. This will be particularly evident when discussing the hypnotizability of alcoholics and drug addicts.

Once again, let's list the four main categories for profiling an individual's hypnotizability:

1. **Psychoanalytic profiling.**
2. **Psychopathological profiling.**
3. **Cultural-ethnic profiling.**
4. **Socio-cultural profiling.**

We will place the greatest emphasis on the first two points, as they are the most significant in our opinion.

3

Psychoanalytic Profiling

In psychoanalytic profiling, it is worth noting the four main profiles of a person's relationships with their parents.

1. **Daddy's and mommy's child**:
   This is a person who loves and accepts both the father and the mother.

2. **Daddy's child, but not mommy's child**:
   This person loves and accepts the father but not the mother.

3. **Mommy's child, but not daddy's child**:
   This person loves and accepts the mother but not the father.

4. **Neither daddy's nor mommy's child**:
   This person, in essence, does not love or accept either the father or the mother.

Daddy's and mommy's child

Individuals with this profile are often highly hypnotizable, at average to high levels, depending on the gender of the hypnotherapist. Trust and love for parental figures become not only psychological but also neurological processes, involving the ability to produce the neurotransmitter oxytocin in the brain, which implies the potential for rapport-building. All patients who underwent therapy with us and corresponded to this profile were hypnotizable and capable of reproducing various trance phenomena.

Daddy's child, but not mommy's child

While working with individuals in this profile, we have found that their ability to enter a hypnotic state is significantly related to their trust in the mother figure. Presumably, this is because the mother is the individual's very first "hypnotherapist," lulling the child to sleep, comforting them during infancy, and being one of the most significant figures from whom the child draws security and peace. When this connection is disrupted, the ability to find an alternative source of balance in the world is also disrupted. We have often observed examples where individuals of this profile initially enter a trance state, but then something seems to interrupt it within them. Deep levels of hypnotic trance are typically less accessible to representatives of this profile. Overall, it should be noted that individuals who are primarily daddy's children do not particularly favor the hypnotic trance; they tend to ignore it, not actively participate in the hypnotic process, and observe others being hypnotized.

Mommy's child, but not daddy's child

On the other hand, mommy's children enjoy the trance state,

and quite strongly at that. They are the most hypnotizable sub-jects among all four psychoanalytic profiles. The vast majority of mommy's children are more willing to surrender control over their consciousness and, at a subconscious level, have a greater desire for the experience of trance. The trance state they experience is usually even deeper than that of Daddy's and Mommy's children. Here, we have made the assumption that the figure of the father in a person's consciousness represents control in various senses of the word. Individuals who love and accept their fathers are generally more willful subjects, which leads us to speculate that the activity of the left prefrontal cortex, associated with a person's volitional qualities and abilities to make independent decisions, may directly relate to the child's psychological relationship with the father figure. Similarly, the activity of the amygdala, anterior and posterior cingulate cortex, brain regions associated with the capacity for empathy and compassion, may be connected to the child's relationship with the mother.

Neither daddy's nor mommy's child

This is the most problematic profile. Subjects with this profile are often only mildly hypnotizable. The lack of emotional connection with the mother greatly hampers their ability to experience the trance state. Moreover, the absence of a connection with the father denies them any opportunities to build their life according to their own desires. Furthermore, it should be added that this profile is the most stagnant and problematic for undergoing psychotherapy. While approaches can eventually be found for other profiles, in this case, any psychotherapeutic interventions are rendered ineffective. The situation changes if it is possible to transform the client's profile into another one, which, in reality, occurs extremely rarely.

4

Imprints of the Perinatal Sphere

The following model of psychoanalytic profiling will be the model proposed by **Stanislav Grof** to describe the psychomotional imprints of the perinatal sphere. This model consists of four **basic perinatal matrices** (**BPM**s) that are analyzed by Grof in terms of their content. However, the analysis of fixations on any perinatal matrices as a capacity for entering into a hypnotic trance has not been conducted, as far as our observations indicate. We will fill this gap by briefly describing these matrices and how their content determines the quality of immersion into a hypnotic state.

BPM-1

The first perinatal matrix, describes almost the entire experience of being in the womb for the infant until the onset of contractions. It is usually associated with a subconscious sense of oceanic bliss, tranquility, and the happiness of unity with the larger world. If the mother did not experience significant stress or emotional turmoil during the entire period of pregnancy, which influences the emotional life of the child, it becomes imprinted on the infant as a favorable state of altered perception. This imprint acts as a beneficial foundation for the ability to enter a hypnotic state. However, experiencing traumatic events during this period does not necessarily imply the opposite effect. Nonetheless, the overall image of an "anxious womb" is likely to disturb profound trust in the world and, specifically, the work of a hypnotherapist.

BPM-2

This perinatal matrix is associated with the experience of the onset of labor, placental rupture, and the initial contractions before cervical dilation. In this matrix, we often encounter the darkest and gloomiest imprints on our psyche. Several factors determine the level of negativity in this matrix. These factors include the level of maternal anxiety at the onset of labor, the duration of the period from the start of contractions to the opening of the cervix, and the general physiological state of the mother during labor. Strong fixation on this matrix can lead to the development of psychopathic or paranoid states in adults, hindering their ability to comfortably experience altered states in general and hypnotic states in particular.

BPM-3

The third perinatal matrix is associated with the process of birth from the beginning of cervical dilation until the moment the baby exits the womb. The passage through the birth canal always leaves a painful imprint on the child. The emotional states experienced by the mother largely determine the child's state, regardless of the difficulties encountered during the process of entering the world. Intense fear, anxiety, and anger in the mother can create the worst imprints, damaging the child's trust in the world throughout childhood and adulthood. Through our analysis of this matrix, we have discovered an interesting correlation: difficult births can sometimes serve as a basis for the child's ability to enter very deep trance states. We explain this phenomenon by speculating that prolonged and painful labors may provoke bursts of activity in an excessive number of opioid receptors in the mother's brain to alleviate the pain of childbirth. This activation may also lead to a deeper suppression of the cerebral cortex, which naturally becomes imprinted on the child. It is worth noting that we have observed this correlation primarily in female hypnotic subjects who have experienced severe physical abuse during childhood. If the abuse did not shape a paranoid personality structure, these subjects often exhibit a high level of hypnotizability. This dependency was not observed as frequently in male hypnotic subjects, possibly because attacks on them from the external world more often result in a need for hyper-control and activation of the cerebral cortex rather than a deep trance state. It should be added that any unexpressed aggression is much easier and more natural to sublimate in an altered state of consciousness. If, for some reason, an individual does not want or cannot express aggression in their normal state of consciousness, one of the optimal outlets for them is immersion into an altered state of consciousness, specifically a hypnotic state. Unfortunately, many individuals resort to alcohol and drugs for self-therapy purposes in order to express hidden aggressive feelings.

BPM-4

According to Stanislav Grof, the fourth perinatal matrix is associated with the period from complete emergence from the mother's womb until approximately five hours after birth. The key element for the harmonious passage of this matrix is the ability of the child to establish physical contact with the mother during this period. This physical contact will play a significant role in the child's ability to establish a psycho-emotional connection with the external world, trust it, and maintain contact. Of course, this factor is just one among many others that influence such states, so we should not attribute absolute influence to this factor. Another significant criterion that requires comment is that if the child does not receive contact with the mother during this time frame, feelings of resentment and aggression can become key imprints within this matrix, negatively affecting a person's ability to enter a hypnotic trance or experience favorable states within it.

5

Psychopathological Profiling

This form of personality profiling provides one of the most detailed maps, enabling us to assess the hypnotizability of individuals. In our work, we will discuss eight fundamental psychopathological profiles and describe how their characteristics influence the level of hypnotizability in a person.

1. **Hysteroid Personality Profile**
   The hysteroid personality profile refers to individuals who exhibit excessive emotionality, attention-seeking behavior, and a tendency to dramatize situations. Such individuals may display high suggestibility and possess a strong need for approval and recognition.

2. **Paranoid Personality Profile**
   The paranoid personality profile is characterized by a pervasive distrust and suspicion of others. These individuals tend to interpret innocent actions as malicious and may struggle to establish rapport and trust with the hypnotist.

3. **Psychopathic Personality Profile**

The psychopathic personality profile refers to individuals who lack empathy, display impulsivity, and engage in manipulative behavior. Due to their resistance to external influences and a tendency to exert control, individuals with this profile may exhibit low hypnotizability.

4. **Obsessive-Compulsive Personality Profile**

The obsessive-compulsive personality profile is associated with perfectionism, rigidity, and a need for control. Individuals with this profile may find it challenging to relax and relinquish control, impacting their ability to enter a hypnotic state.

5. **Schizoid Personality Profile**

The schizoid personality profile describes individuals characterized by social withdrawal, emotional detachment, and introspection. These individuals may encounter difficulties establishing rapport with the hypnotist and may exhibit low hypnotizability.

6. **Epileptoid Personality Profile**

The epileptoid personality profile is linked to emotional instability, impulsivity, and intense emotional reactions. Individuals with this profile may demonstrate heightened hypnotizability due to their susceptibility to emotional states.

7. **Schizophrenic Personality Profile**

The schizophrenic personality profile involves disturbances in perception, thought processes, and social functioning. The level of hypnotizability may vary among individuals with this profile, depending on the severity of their symptoms and their ability to maintain focus.

8. **Manic-Depressive Personality Profile** (Bipolar)
   The manic-depressive personality profile is characterized by extreme mood swings, ranging from manic episodes of high energy to depressive episodes of low mood. The hypnotizability of individuals with this profile may fluctuate depending on their current mood state.

All the manifestations of these psychopathological profiles can be differentiated into **three levels of intensity**:

1. **Accentuated Level**:
   Pathology is in its incipient stage and does not significantly impact social adequacy. It merely gives the personality a specific direction.

2. **Neurotic Level**:
   Pathology significantly impairs social adaptation.

3. **Psychotic Level**:
   The ability for social adaptation is almost completely disrupted by various forms of symptom manifestation.

By understanding these profiles and their intensity levels, we gain insights into an individual's susceptibility to hypnosis, enabling us to tailor therapeutic approaches accordingly.

6

Hysteroid Personality Profile

As the starting point for developing this profiling model, we took the illness of hysteria and its less pathological form of expression, known as hysteroid (demonstrative) accentuation. As we mentioned, early hypnotherapists discovered that women suffering from hysteria were extremely hypnotizable. Hysteria was initially considered a predominantly female disorder. Hippocrates believed that hysteria was a manifestation of the "wandering womb." Plato stated that hysteria afflicts women who are unable to conceive. Ancient Greeks often recommended marrying young girls as a quick remedy for hysteria. It is also mentioned that in Ancient Greece, methods involving Dionysian practices, such as wine and orgies, were sometimes used to treat hysteria. We will not assert the correctness of the ancient Greeks, but we can assume that these methods may have provided temporary improvement while likely worsening the condition in the long term. In medieval Europe, women suffering from hysteria were often accused of witchcraft by the Inquisition and burned at the stake. It is worth noting that hysterics are highly hypnotizable, and we are convinced that if a hysteric woman is suggested to be possessed by an evil force, she will eventually "play out" this possession. Early psychiatrists considered hysteria the mother of imitation since they noticed that hysterical individuals were capable of displaying almost all the symptoms characteristic of other illnesses in their behavior. Even in the 19th century, the treatment of hysteria did not differ significantly from the Dionysian methods of the ancient Greeks. Physicians in Britain, France, and some other European countries could suggest clitoral massage as a therapy for hysterical patients.

In the late 19th century, sets for "self-massage" even started being sold in British pharmacies. As some contemporary psychiatrists write, these are the milestones in the history of medicine that today's medical professionals might feel ashamed of. We don't know about shame, but when we share this historical information with our students during courses on psychopathology and psychotherapy, we mainly observe laughter.

Here we can clearly trace a peculiar dependence. Early psychiatrists primarily treated hysteroid women with massages and hypnosis. They witnessed the complete compliance of their patients with their suggestions. Orgasm and deep hypnotic states share similarities in their neurophysiological processes. The deeper the trance state, the lower the activity in the cerebral cortex of the brain.

Understanding the hysteroid personality profile is essential in the context of psychopathological profiling. Individuals with this profile tend to exhibit attention-seeking behavior, dramatic expressions of emotions, and a strong desire for recognition. They may display high hypnotizability due to their inclination toward suggestibility. It is important to note that the term "hysteroid" is used here to describe a specific accentuation or emphasis within the personality structure rather than a clinical diagnosis of hysteria. By studying this profile and its influence on hypnotizability, we gain valuable insights into therapeutic approaches that can be tailored to individuals with such characteristics.

It is crucial to approach the historical treatment methods mentioned with critical analysis and acknowledge the progress made in medical ethics and evidence-based practices. Contemporary understanding and treatment of psychopathology, including the hysteroid personality profile, emphasize the importance of comprehensive assessment, evidence-based interventions, and a compassionate therapeutic relationship. By integrating psychological theories, clinical expertise, and ethical considerations, we strive to provide effective and ethical care to individuals with various psychopathological profiles.

Working with patients who exhibited prominent symptoms of hysteria or hysteric accentuation, we have confirmed that this symptom provides an ideal foundation for hypnosis. Hysteroid patients not only more frequently enter very deep altered states of consciousness, but their style of entering a hypnotic state is often extravagant, vivid, and memorable. These are truly the moments that are easily remembered and stay with us for years.

Let us provide some vivid examples from our practice. One of our students, clearly possessing hysteroid accentuation, had the ability to enter a state of hypnosis simply by touching her forehead and giving the command, "Sleep!" Within a couple of seconds of this, her body would completely relax and become "gelatinous." If she was seated in this state, she would eventually attempt to fall to the floor.

Once, she participated in an evening hypnosis class that lasted from 5:00 PM to 9:00 PM. At the end of the class, we took her for a hypnotic session and easily and quickly induced her into a hypnotic state. We suggested to her that she would forget the past four hours and that upon awakening from the hypnotic trance, she would firmly believe that she had just arrived for the evening session. We also suggested that she fully remember the forgotten time by the next morning.

Then we commanded her to awaken from her hypnotic sleep. She looked at us in surprise, then at the other participants in the group, and finally out of the window, where it was already dark. She was shocked by the sudden change in lighting outside and then commented with surprise, "I have a strange feeling as if everything has already happened." For several hours after the group session, fragments of the lost time would emerge for her. By the following morning, all the memories had returned. This was one of the most vivid examples in our practice of selective hypnotic amnesia.

It was impossible to reproduce the phenomena of catalepsy and levitation of the hands in her case, as her body in trance was always "gelatinous." Suggestions did not help in this case. In the hypnotic trance state, she perfectly executed suggestions to open her eyes and see things that were not there, meaning she experienced positive hallucinations.

In one of the seminars on Ericksonian hypnosis, while in a hypnotic trance, we suggested to her that she would easily enter a hypnotic trance upon hearing the key phrase "Stormy Petrel." Then we induced amnesia regarding the suggestion, brought her out of trance, placed her in the center of the auditorium (with a young man standing behind her to catch her if she fell), and said the suggested word. Her eyes began to close, and her body started to slump downward. When we repeated the key phrase, she collapsed to the ground. The young man caught her just in time. This example clearly demonstrates the phenomenal level of her hypnotic susceptibility.

Another student, also possessing hysteroid accentuation, was highly suggestible, just like the previous one. It only took a couple of words, sometimes just a touch to her forehead, and she would already be deep in a hypnotic trance.

Her main difference from the previous student was her motor disinhibition during the process of trance induction. A single touch to her hand and lifting it upwards would create a stable catalepsy of the hand. Moreover, it was possible to quickly induce this form of hypnotic catalepsy even when she was not in a typical hypnotic trance state. We could induce catalepsy in both her hands and legs simultaneously during the trance. Furthermore, the catalepsy of the hands would frequently transition naturally into levitation. In other words, the hands would smoothly move in the air and live their own peculiar life.

It was with her that we easily and naturally created the phenomenon of catalepsy of the entire body, where the body acquires wax-like flexibility and pliability, assumes a stable standing position, and then, with the help of an assistant, the hypnotized body is placed on the backs of chairs. The upper part of the back on one chair and the lower part of the legs on another chair. We could place up to five metal office chairs on her abdomen during this procedure, and her body remained stable.

Additionally, she exhibited excellent positive and negative hallucination phenomena during hypnosis sessions. The phenomena of hypermnesia, amnesia, anesthesia, analgesia, taste illusions, and other phenomena were easily achieved. It is worth noting an interesting aspect of her profile. She almost completely denied her own sexuality and had no desire to engage in any sexual relationships. This persisted until she turned 25. We do not possess information about what happened after the age of 25.

It would be logical to assume that her hyper-hypnotizability was somehow related to sexual repression. However, it is not that simple. The previous hypnotic subject we described, who was highly suggestible, did not exhibit sexual abstinence at all.

All the clients with hysteroid accentuation who participated in our hypnosis sessions frequently and effortlessly achieved a somnambulistic trance state, and the manifestations of trance were particularly vivid and remarkable.

By employing elementary behavior analysis, it was possible to identify manifestations of hysteroid accentuation in clients, thereby suggesting a higher level of hypnotizability.

Key characteristics of hysteroid behavior:

1. Constant attention-seeking behavior.
2. Desire to actively participate in discussions.
3. Willingness to publicly discuss personal aspects of their life and the lives of others.
4. If the hysteroid individual is female, their behavior is often sexualized, especially around men.
5. Display of intense emotions.
6. Problems with self-control, willpower, and goal-setting.
7. Occasional tactlessness and unethical behavior.
8. Hysteroid men have a high likelihood of substance abuse and alcohol dependence.
9. Frequent lying.

10. Inclination towards fantasy.
11. Desire for public engagement and exposure.
12. Strong craving for public approval.
13. High probability of infidelity towards their sexual partner.
14. Often characterized by an attention-grabbing appearance and clothing.
15. Tendency to engage in unexpected, sometimes shocking actions.

By observing a person for just a couple of hours, many of these criteria will begin to manifest in their behavior. In our opinion, individuals fitting this profile are ideal for demonstrating various phenomena of hypnotic trance.

Assessment of Hypnotic Susceptibility Profile Characteristics:

1. Very high hypnotic susceptibility
2. Rapid induction into a hypnotic state
3. Almost complete absence of resistance to the hypnotherapist
4. Exaggeration of hypnotic effects
5. Exaggeration of therapeutic effects
6. Deeper and faster immersion into a hypnotic state in public settings
7. High risk of erotic transference onto the psychotherapist
8. Strong short-term and weak long-term therapeutic effect

7

Paranoid Personality Profile

Paranoid personalities are no less intriguing in hypnotherapy than hysteric ones, as they represent the diametrical opposite in their ability to enter a state of hypnotic trance. The paranoid profile is one of the least hypnotizable profiles in our model. Paranoid individuals have existed throughout the history of humanity. A paranoid personality organizes their thinking in a way that constantly seeks to perceive threats to themselves, their family, their city, their country, and so on. To some extent, a paranoid individual lives in their own world, where they believe that their surroundings intend to make them victims. In our opinion, there are six main types of paranoia that can actively develop in a person's mind.

1. **Paranoia of rumors**:
   The person believes that others speak negatively about them, insult them behind their backs, consider them bad, insignificant, immoral, and so on.

2. **Physical harm paranoia**:

The person believes that they may be beaten, maimed, injured, or subjected to any other form of physical harm.

3. **Sexual harm paranoia**:
This type of paranoia is predominantly found in women. They believe that they are in danger of being raped, seduced, or sexually exploited. They develop a conviction that men are only interested in one thing.

4. **Theft paranoia**:
These individuals have persistent thoughts that their apartment will be burglarized, their personal belongings will be stolen, or that someone will deceive them in order to gain material benefits. They develop a worldview in which financially motivated people surround them, willing to do anything for a penny, and so on.

5. **Social harm paranoia**:
The main focus here is on conspiracies aimed at demoting them from a position, firing them from work, blocking their career advancement, and so on.

6. **Betrayal by friends and infidelity paranoia**:
Intrusive thoughts about being abandoned by loved ones.

These are the primary manifestations of paranoia, which can actively occur within an individual's mind.

From our experience, the majority of different cases of paranoia in individuals can be classified into one of these six categories. Sometimes paranoia remains in a passive form, where a person contemplates the world but refrains from taking any significant actions based on their thoughts. However, the stronger the paranoia,

the greater the desire to transition into an active form, where the paranoid individual, instead of waiting for an attack, becomes the attacker themselves. They inflict harm upon people they suspect of conspiracy and betray their partners after inventing the belief that the partner has already betrayed them.

The main distinction from paranoid schizophrenia is that a paranoid individual does not experience hallucinations or sensory illusions. Everything happens within the framework of an ordinary cognitive process that remains confined to their mind.

Naturally, the constant fixation of one's thoughts on potential danger keeps the individual in a state of both emotional and muscular tension. The cortex of the cerebral hemispheres is constantly hyperactive, causing significant difficulties for the person to naturally enter altered states of consciousness, particularly hypnosis. Over the years, we have observed how individuals with a paranoid personality accent or suffering from full-blown paranoia are capable of reacting to the process of inducing a hypnotic trance.

Trust issues typically arise at the beginning of hypnotic work, where the patient expresses numerous negative assumptions and concerns about what they may expect in the trance state. Men may often worry about whether the hypnotic trance will negatively affect them. Women, on the other hand, are more frequently plagued by sexual paranoia, fearing that they will be helpless with a hypnotherapist who may do whatever they desire. Such fantasies can sometimes be found in the imaginations of female clients.

Regarding the impact on states in the context of hypnotic induction, paranoia can be divided into deep, true paranoia and superficial, hysterical paranoia. Deep, true paranoia primarily affects neurophysiological processes, interrupting any attempts to enter a trance state with active cognitive processes and physical tension. The client may already be consciously convinced that nothing threatens them, but old paranoid defense mechanisms will hinder the entry into an altered state of consciousness in any attempts by the hypnotherapist. Let me provide an example.

About five years ago, we conducted a workshop dedicated to hypnotic suggestion in an anti-café in the city. The owner of the establishment, who provided the venue for the event, participated in the class. In the final part of the seminar, we demonstrated a session of group induction into a hypnotic trance, during which anyone in the group could immerse themselves in an altered state. At the end of the trance session, participants provided feedback regarding the states they experienced during the hypnotic induction. When it was the turn of the establishment owner, she commented the following: "I sat with my eyes closed, and thoughts kept racing through my head that while we were sitting like this, you were rummaging through our bags." In this case, we clearly observe paranoia related to theft and causing material harm.

Analyzing the causes of such states in clients, we found either situations where the person had been repeatedly robbed in the past, resulting in a significantly increased level of anxiety regarding the safety of their belongings, or the person themselves had once been a thief and is now simply projecting their past actions onto others, unwilling to remember and acknowledge their own deeds. When it comes to sexual paranoia among women, the situation differs slightly.

If the first criterion remains similar to the previous one, and if a woman has experienced sexual violence, attempted sexual violence, or aggressive sexual harassment, then the main second criterion will be paranoia induced by suggestion. For example, it could stem from the mother or grandmother in the woman's childhood, where constant ideas were instilled in the family that the image of a man is that of a lustful animal who only wants "one thing." Sometimes we can observe combinations of both the first and second criteria.

We made another very interesting observation regarding the process of hypnotization as well as other practices of altered states of consciousness. It is inherent for people to project those feelings that they usually repress or wish to repress in their everyday lives. During the anticipation of hypnosis and often during the first hypnosis session, these repressed products begin to actively enter the conscious sphere. As a result, individuals may experience aggressive, anxious, phobic, sexualized emotions, feelings of helplessness, sadness, and so on. However, if a person does not possess a paranoid personality accent, these symptoms usually subside after the first hypnosis session and do not return. In contrast, individuals with a paranoid personality accent may remain fixated on negative experiences for an indefinite amount of time. Sometimes, suppressed negative emotions may somatize during the first hypnosis session. For example, a strong headache may arise, which can persist for several hours after the hypnosis session. In all cases we observed, the initial somatization never recurred during subsequent trance sessions.

Superficial hysterical paranoia often manifests as exaggerated anxiety regarding what to expect during the hypnotic state.

Clients express their concerns, display hesitancy, and approach everything with caution. However, if the trance session can be initiated, these anxieties usually transform into a passive background form, allowing the client to enter a light or even moderate level of hypnotic trance.

In the vast majority of cases, a paranoid personality accent makes hypnotherapy minimally productive or unproductive altogether. Occasionally, prolonged verbal therapy can reduce paranoid reactions, enabling the utilization of hypnotic practices during later stages of psychotherapy.

Key characteristics of the paranoid type:

- Distrust
- Suspiciousness
- Fixation on negative outcomes of events
- Inability to acknowledge one's own mistakes
- Interpreting all life events according to a paranoid world-view
- Anxiety
- Unconscious provocation by the environment to engage in negative actions
- Hypochondria
- Pessimism
- Persecutory delusions
- Paranoid fantasies

Assessment of the hypnability profile:

- Low or minimal level of hypnotizability
- Almost complete inability to engage in the hypnotic process, particularly during initial attempts
- If trance does occur, it is often superficial and not deep
- Underestimation of the power of hypnotic effects by the patient
- Underestimation of the therapeutic effects
- Public induction of trance may increase patient discomfort
- Risk of aggressive transference onto the psychotherapist.

8

Psychopathic Personality Profile

There are a wide variety of manifestations of psychopathic behavior. Behind psychopathic behavior, certain **key personality
characteristics** are often present. Let's list them:

1. Inability to experience guilt, shame, or embarrassment.
2. Disregard for morality in various forms.
3. Almost complete absence of fear.
4. Almost complete inability to sympathize, empathize, or
   show empathy.
5. Almost complete absence of depressive and anxious symptoms.
6. Living day by day without significant future planning.
7. Narcissism, selfishness, and self-centeredness.
8. High level of Machiavellianism (life principle: "the ends
   justify the means").
9. Often, high levels of communication skills.
10. Often, a high level of personal charm.
11. Pleasure derived from causing suffering to others in
    various forms.

Naturally, the intensity of these manifestations can vary greatly, ranging from microscopic expressions where the psychopath simply derives pleasure from causing relatively minor emotional pain to severe forms of physical and sexual violence.

Separate from typical true psychopathy is sexual psychopathy, where an individual simply has a need to engage in deviant sexual acts, sometimes involving violence and harm to others and sometimes without it. This can include fetishes, BDSM, voyeurism, exhibitionism, pedophilia, necrophilia, and more. Various forms of sexual psychopathy may not necessarily be sadistic in nature, where an individual derives sexual pleasure specifically from the process of strangling a sexual partner, but masochistic, where there is a strong desire for certain ritual forms of violence to be performed on the individual themselves, resulting in sexual gratification. In our work, we will not delve deeply into the topic of sexual psychopathy, as it deserves separate and detailed attention. For now, we will simply outline its general contours to link it to the theme of the patient's hypnotizability in the process of hypnosis.

Sometimes psychopathy takes on a hysteroid, demonstrative accent when a person seeks to appear unfeeling, narcissistic, and walking over corpses—a "genius of our time." But in reality, we will see that beneath the mask hides a frightened individual.

Based on our experience, **true psychopaths are almost entirely unhypnotizable**. Problems with hypnotizing individuals of this profile can be even more pronounced than with individuals of the paranoid profile. Sexual psychopaths, without extreme forms of manifestation, can vary in their response to hypnotic suggestion, ranging from strong resistance to complete compliance, similar to hysteroid personalities. These changes, in our opinion, vary according to the psychoanalytic profile of the individual.

Based on our observations, demonstrative psychopaths are more often hypnotizable at a low or moderate level. Let us provide examples to further analyze representatives of this profile and its variations.

We will not describe severe forms of psychopathy, only those that we interpret as accentuated forms.

A 38-year-old female patient came with a very interesting request related to her husband and several lovers in different countries who are competing for her hand. She sleeps with each of them in turn, and she enjoys it, but she is troubled by the fact that she enjoys it. It is worth mentioning that her request was extremely original.

During the conversation, it became clear that she completely lacks a sense of guilt for her relationships with men. As she said, she constantly has 2-3 men in her life, and these are not just lovers but full-fledged relationships. Fortunately, they are all scattered across different countries. In most of these relationships, she does not experience complete sexual satisfaction, which often leads her to engage in autoeroticism. She does not feel the need to choose one particular man. This displays a symptom closely resembling nymphomania.

She mentioned that she collects rings from men who have asked her to marry them. She often brings these relationships to the point of marriage and then runs away. When she was 18 years old, she started a relationship with a 26-year-old college director where she was studying. The man was in love with her and, as she said, carried her in his hands. They planned their wedding. However, she did not show up for the wedding and instead went to another man, with whose help she had an abortion. She got pregnant by the next man and had an abortion with him as well. She then met a man who became her husband and the father of her child.

Her attitude towards men is devoid of sentimentality and is seen as a means to satisfy her sexual needs. She denies feeling guilt for any of her actions. She regards psychotherapy as an interesting game, much like any psychopath. In this case, we observe a combination of true and sexual psychopathy. On the one hand, true psychopathy blocks almost all natural entry points into a hypnotic state. On the other hand, sexual uninhibitedness can significantly contribute to the presence of a need for deep unconscious states. In this case, true psychopathic accentuation predominated.

The patient became interested in hypnosis practice. She was very nervous before the session, as if she couldn't find her place. During attempts to hypnotize her, her body experienced spasms, and almost every muscle tensed, even though she did not make any conscious effort to do so. Her reactions to the hypnotherapist somewhat resembled those of paranoid personalities, but without any explicit expectation of harm to herself. After intentionally closing her eyes at the request of the hypnotherapist, she began to think that the hypnotherapist was looking at her face very intently. The tension in her body increased, and she abruptly opened her eyes. This happened several times during the session.

The psychopath's ego faced a direct attack on its defense mechanisms. Psychopaths constantly suppress the sense of guilt for their actions, but the process of suppression requires constant energy expenditure, manifested in the body as fixed muscle tension. If a psychopath tries hypnotic influence, it relaxes their muscular framework, connecting them to a sense of guilt, which is painful for them. The only way to prevent this is to do anything to avoid it. We have discovered similar reactions in true psychopaths to Stanislav Grof's holotropic breathwork. Most other profiles can immerse themselves in interesting and vivid states of consciousness using this method in psychotherapeutic work, but true psychopaths often experience intense suffering and usually terminate the session as unbearable.

It should be noted that psychopathic personalities often replace natural trance states with substances like heroin, cocaine, and marijuana. However, not all of them do so.

So let's summarize true psychopathy. Patients in this category are among the most unhypnotizable individuals. However, such patients rarely seek therapy, and if they do, they perceive it as an interesting pastime rather than a psychotherapeutic process. When you tell these people directly to their faces that they don't want to change their way of life, they sincerely confirm this belief and continue attending psychotherapy sessions. A natural question arises: why? The answer here is almost unequivocal. The world of a psychopath is a world of aggressor and victim, and it is vital for them to continue playing the role of the aggressor with all their might. At the first opportunity, a psychopath will try to assume the role of the victim towards the therapist, if successful. If they realize that they are unlikely to succeed, they leave psychotherapy and return to their usual activities.

The situation may be somewhat different with pure sexual psychopaths. Sexual psychopathy manifests itself in various forms, and we have not had the opportunity to work with many of them using hypnotic suggestion. Our observations indicate that certain sexual perversions performed in privacy or with mutually agreed-upon partners can significantly influence the depth of hypnotizability, sometimes enabling individuals to reach ultra-deep trance states.

Unfortunately, in our opinion, the overwhelming majority of psychopaths and sexual deviants do not voluntarily seek psychotherapists, making it genuinely challenging to assemble a comprehensive clinical picture in such cases. Let's provide an example of a case of sexual psychopathy.

A 27-year-old female patient during the course of therapy. From childhood until the age of 18, she regularly experienced aggressive violence. Her father would regularly beat her, grab her by the hair, slam her head against the tiles, and humiliate her. She always assumed a passive victim position towards her father. Menstruation began at the age of 15. Her sexuality remained inactive until the age of 21. At 21, she encountered a young man with whom she had a relationship for a while. Then, in the woods, according to her comments, she had sexual intercourse coerced by him. After that, she broke up with him, and for the following 3 years, she displayed strong sexual uninhibitedness in her behavior. She engaged in relationships with dozens of men, whom she could simply find on the street and bring home for one-time sexual encounters. She doesn't remember the names of most of these people. During this period and subsequently, she exhibited a strong attraction to BDSM in her sexual relationships, assuming a passive position. After these three years, her sexuality somewhat calmed down, and she found a somewhat regular sexual partner with whom she had sex several times a year. She also found a married man whom she fell in love with and continuously attempted to win over from his wife, a pursuit she continued for many years. At times, she felt the need to find a BDSM "dominator" who could engage in perverted forms of intercourse with her. As she commented, she experienced special pleasure when performing fellatio with such men, "until tears, pain, and vomiting." This particular form of sex provided her with intense sexual and psychoemotional release. During psychotherapy sessions, she directly referred to herself as a sexual psychopath, expressing her enjoyment and eagerly describing her sexual exploits in detail. At the same time, she claimed to love only one man, who happened to be married. She wanted to marry him and have a child with him.

Her reactions to hypnotic trance were some of the deepest we have seen. Any form of hypnotic induction quickly and easily induced an altered state of consciousness in her. She was capable of delving into deep, unconscious levels of hypnotic trance. She could generate many, but not all, hypnotic phenomena. For example, she experienced difficulties reproducing the cataleptic arm phenomenon since her body relaxed at the deepest level of hypnosis, becoming jelly-like. Encountering similar bodily reactions in some patients on multiple occasions, we named this phenomenon the "limp body syndrome" and the "limp arm syndrome," in which any form given to the body or its parts is lost and dissolves. During trance sessions, she generated a multitude of meaningful associations, which distinguished her from other hypnotic subjects.

During the process of working with holotropic breathwork, she also displayed phenomenal results. While other partici-pants sometimes required at least 15–20 minutes to experience initial changes in their state of consciousness through intensive breathing, it only took her about five minutes for a true "psychedelic" revolution to unfold within her. She had visions of her past incarnations, associations with animals, and so on. During a holotropic breathwork session, she would frequently pause every 5 minutes, grab a pen and notebook, and record fragments of her journey into the depths of the unconscious. We rarely witnessed such extraordinary abilities to recreate the depth and intensity of trance states in anyone else.

It is worth adding some other elements to her profile. In all other areas of life, she is a very kind and compassionate person, capable of empathy towards others. She adores pets and enjoys participating in volunteer movements that aid others during challenging periods of their lives.

Based on our observations, individuals with a sexual psychopathy profile similar to the example described above tend to have a significant predisposition to immerse themselves in very deep trance states. We explain this phenomenon by the fact that this category of individuals extensively trains the cortex of their cerebral hemispheres to temporarily disconnect, allowing more ancient archaic brain structures to become active for a certain period of time. By the way, the situation with hypnotizability among alcoholics is similar to that of accentuated sexual psychopaths.

Assessment of hypnotizability characteristics within the profile:

- Minimal, weak, and moderate levels of hypnotizability are possible, depending on the orientation of psychopathy.
- Hyper-hypnotizability is possible in cases of sexual psychopathy.
- The trance state is never truly deep.
- There is a risk of deception in the patient's feedback

regarding the hypnotic process.

- The ability to manifest only certain minor hypnotic phenomena.
- Almost complete absence of psychotherapeutic effect.

9

Obsessive-Compulsive Personality Profile

Obsessive-compulsive personality disorder manifests in various forms of obsessive thinking and subsequent ritualistic behavior. The thinking triggers personal anxiety, which can only be reduced or alleviated by performing a specific sequence of actions. For example, a person leaves home and then has the obsessive thought that they didn't lock the door. They return to the door, check the lock, confirm that it's locked, move away from the house, and once again experience the same worry that the door might not be securely closed, prompting them to return to the lock. In mild cases of OCD, the number of repetitions may be 2-3, while in severe cases, it can reach dozens. We knew a patient who had such obsessiveness and attempted to cope with it in a unique way by recording the process of closing the door on their mobile phone. When they experienced anxiety upon leaving the house, they simply played the video on their phone, watched the recording, and temporarily calmed down.

The ritualistic form of OCD can take various forms, such

as arranging objects symmetrically in a room, tidying up the space, checking electrical appliances to ensure they are unplugged, or verifying that the gas on the stove is turned off, among others. The unfulfilled need for compulsive action always leads to an increase in anxiety levels, and sooner or later, the patient "breaks down." Attempts to exert voluntary control over the behavior often yield no results. Moreover, the patient is fully aware of the absurdity and genuine uselessness of such actions. Sometimes, the ritualistic behavior takes on a mythological character as the patient tries to attribute special meanings to their actions. They may invent their own signs or follow popular beliefs.

One of our patients with OCD, when he entered our office and saw that the books on the shelf were not arranged thematically, asked us for permission to rearrange them. Then, as his gaze fell upon the certificates hanging on the wall, he noticed that some of them were not perfectly level and expressed the desire to adjust them.

The key emotion for individuals with OCD is guilt. The compulsion to align, correct, and check everything reflects an experience where something was not done well enough. Symbolically, the compulsion brings the person back to the traumatic experience and attempts to complete or redo its content.

From a psychoanalytic perspective, we have found that the severity of the disorder is closely related to the patient's relationship with the father figure. OCD patients often view the father figure as flawed and unworthy of emulation. The aforementioned patient, who obsessively wanted to adjust the books and certificates in our office, was a former priest. He was a very kind and balanced individual with a vast knowledge base.

His father was a highly aggressive and unpredictable person.

OCD patients approach any form of psychotherapy very cautiously, sometimes perceiving it as a ritual to relieve their sense of guilt, which is not always fully recognized. This applies to hypnotic practice as well. Their need for everything to be correct and harmonious is so great that it influences neurological processes in the context of hypnotic induction.

Trans-states usually have a moderate-to-deep level of depth. Processes of understanding and reevaluation unfold actively during trance. As for hypnotic phenomena, what we have observed is that catalepsy of the hand, levitation, anesthesia, and analgesia are excellently formed. More complex phenomena, such as positive and negative hallucinations, are less effectively formed.

Another significant value of trance for individuals with OCD tendencies is that, unlike hysteroids and sexual psychopaths, they possess a special sense of moderation in reproducing trance phenomena, never exaggerating their effects, in our opinion. In many ways, in terms of the experience of hypnotic trance, they resemble epileptoid-accentuated personalities, which we will discuss briefly later.

Additionally, it is worth noting that when applying the method of holotropic breathing developed by Stanislav Grof, we observe a relatively rapid and deep immersion into an altered state. Simply participating regularly in the process of trance induction can significantly alleviate anxiety states and reduce the intensity of compulsive actions.

Key characteristics of the paranoid OCD type include:

- Obsessive thoughts, actions, and reminiscences (visual memories).
- Perfectionism.
- Tendency toward closure of gestalt.
- Inability to stop obsessions.
- Increased anxiety when unable to complete tasks.
- Ritualization of actions.
- Conscious or hidden feelings of guilt.

Assessment of hypnability profile characteristics:

- Strong or maximum level of hypnotizability.
- Very high need for trance states. Unlike hysteroid profiles, the phenomena are more 'realistic'.
- Working with trance without exaggeration or understatement of the trance effect.
- Working with trance without exaggeration or understatement of the psychotherapeutic effect.
- Strong short-term and long-term psychotherapeutic effects.

Recommended Therapy Service for OCD

- Quick client-counselor matching
- Licensed professionals only
- Flexible subscription options that fit your budget
- Free counselor switching

10

Schizoid Personality Profile

A person with a schizoid personality profile is emotionally cold and absorbed in their thoughts about the world and their fantasies. They avoid emotional relationships with others. Ernst Kretschmer, a German psychiatrist, referred to schizoids as 'Friends of Books and Nature.' Schizoids lack affective resonance with other people. They are unable to effectively express their own emotions and understand the emotions of others. They may not attach much importance to social norms and live by their own rules, but they do not disrupt social order and are often perceived by others as 'not of this world.'

The main characteristics of schizoid disorder may include the following:

- Emotional coldness.
- Difficulties in expressing emotions.
- Difficulties in understanding the emotions of others.
- Need for solitary activities.
- Stiff and robotic gait.
- Monotonous and cold voice.

- Almost complete lack of eye contact during communication.
- Inclination towards highly intellectual activities.
- Wearing peculiar clothing.
- Ignoring other people's problems (the 'tree and glass' symptom).
- Narcissism.
- Self-sufficiency.
- Either no friends or very few (often just one close friend for schizoids).
- Strong emotional vulnerability that schizoids try not to show to anyone.
- Dislike of sports and physical practices in general.

Naturally, all the mentioned symptoms can occur at different levels of intensity. However, they most often form a cohesive and comprehensive profile.

Based on our observations, individuals with a schizoid personality are often resentful towards the maternal figure in their family, and less frequently towards the father, especially if the mother assumes a more masculine role in the family. The inability to establish a meaningful emotional connection with a significant figure in the family deeply wounds the schizoid, causing them to withdraw into themselves.

In childhood or adolescence, the schizoid learns that they can mostly rely only on themselves and that, essentially, they do not need anyone else. As schizoids tend to become self-sufficient much earlier than others, thanks to their considerable cognitive abilities, their self-esteem develops and they display it in extravagant ways, further complicating their already challenging emotional relationships with others.

In childhood, schizoids are often rejected by their peers and become outcasts. However, as they mature and develop their personalities, schizoids become sought after in various groups due to their professional qualities, thoughtfulness, perseverance, and original creative ideas. It is during this time that they gradually gain more and more opportunities for emotional contact with other people. If circumstances align favorably, they can gradually emerge from their cocoon. However, strong stress and negative emotions in relationships can easily pull them back in.

On the surface, it may seem that a schizoid personality is resistant to hypnosis, but that is not the case at all. Hypnotic work can reveal surprising possibilities for psychotherapy, especially when the schizoid profile is combined with a paranoid aspect. If the paranoid aspect is not involved, hypnotic work can be quite effective in therapy.

Empathy toward the surrounding world is greatly blocked in schizoids due to their past emotional traumas. Their inability to empathize with others is a form of aggression. The more aggression they harbor towards the world, the greater their need for dissociation and detachment. This is how the schizoid seeks revenge against the world, to some extent destroying themselves in the process. Furthermore, the stronger their aggression, the more peculiar their world of illusions and fantasies becomes.

However, if a person capable of sharing their often strange reality appears and consistently demonstrates loyalty to their world through actions, a 'miracle' can occur, and the schizoid may accept that person as their own. This person doesn't necessarily have to be another schizoid, although that is possible. Cooperation can also occur with individuals of other profiles. A similar structure of relationships can emerge in an alliance with a psychotherapist. Through the therapeutic process and their professional skills, the therapist establishes rapport with the patient. With increasing trust, the therapist can become the schizoid's 'sole friend.' This is beneficial as the schizoid gains the opportunity to relearn trust in the world, to speak about their feelings, and to express them freely. However, this often requires time—sometimes months.

During the initial stages of psychotherapy, patients with this profile avoid eye contact, may appear peculiar, and often complain about difficulties in forming friendly and intimate relationships. The sexual sphere is almost always problematic for schizoids. They either completely deny its existence or sometimes settle for autoeroticism. Some of them engage in sexual relationships not because they desire them but, as they say, 'to not stand out too much from others.' However, this is rare. In this case, the depth of the schizoid accent in their personality plays a significant role. Naturally, the deeper the symptomatology, the poorer the prognosis. Sexual connections may be absent until the ages of 25, 30, 35, or even longer. The first sexual experience for a schizoid can end in both emotional and sexual failure and can completely close them off from intimacy for many years.

With a psychotherapist, a schizoid can eventually open up and engage effectively, participating in hypnotherapy sessions that yield significant results in terms of change and trans-formation. However, the schizoid often desires to turn the psychotherapist into a friend and almost a family member, attempting to replace key social roles. The dynamics of this process can vary greatly and are highly individual.

When discussing the schizoid's ability to participate in

hypnotherapy sessions, it is important to mention that initially, the schizoid may exhibit reactions similar to those of a highly ungainable individual. Their tendency towards hyper-rationalization and criticism, resulting in hyperactivity of the cerebral cortex, does not dissipate quickly. However, with each session, deeper levels can be reached, and over time, an individual who initially seemed almost entirely ungainable may begin to exhibit phenomena accessible to highly hypnotizable individuals. Naturally, as hypnotizability improves, we have observed numerous enhancements in social communication skills. The unveiling in hypnotic trance could become a metaphor for the unveiling in social communication.

For instance, one patient with a schizoid profile initially complained about not being able to grasp social rhythms, constantly saying inappropriate things that irritated colleagues at work. Throughout a year of regular therapy, he participated in multiple hypnotherapy sessions, continuously discovering something new while in trance. Over this period, his social communication with colleagues and friends underwent slow but steady changes. More emotions emerged in his communication, and he became less afraid of being rejected, becoming more socially active. By the end of the year, he could already recount instances where he became the life of the party at work, easily engaging in humor and philosophical discussions on various topics. Of course, therapy was not without its challenges, but the overall trajectory was positive.

We have observed a fascinating phenomenon regarding how schizoid individuals can integrate trance experiences into their behavior. Some of them, after a series of hypnosis sessions, may begin to attempt to recreate the state of trance and certain hypnotic phenomena themselves. For example, one young man, after experiencing catalepsy of the entire body several times (a phenomenon where the subject's body is placed between the backs of chairs after catalepsy is induced), started asking us, "Can I achieve this on my own at home?" Another patient began sharing that deep trance states with vivid and colorful sensory presentations started occurring to him at home while he was engaged in various activities. This same patient started integrating the phenomenon of analog body signaling, which we had repeatedly created in our hypnosis sessions (more details about this phenomenon will be provided in the chapter dedicated to hypnotic phenomena), into his everyday life. Another patient started attempting to induce hypnotic states by himself at home. Here we see that the overall strategy towards the world, where the schizoid attempts to do everything independently, disregarding social connections, is sometimes nearly unshakeable.

Evaluation of hypnotizability characteristics within the profile:

- At the beginning of therapy, a minimal level of hypnotizability may be present, but as rapport develops, experiences of heightened hypnotic responses become possible.
- Initial attempts at inducing a trance may be unsuccessful.
- With each hypnotic induction, a positive trend and deeper level of hypnotic trance can be observed.
- The hypnotic trance itself teaches the schizoid individual a sense of connection with the world.
- The act of inducing the hypnotic state itself is more therapeutic than the specific suggestions given during the trance state.

11

Epileptoid Personality Profile

The epileptoid personality is emotionally "hot" in contrast to the cold schizoid personality. It is characterized by emotional outbursts, often accompanied by motor activity. While working with epileptoids, we have found an adequate metaphor in the strategy of relating to the world: the "guilty criminal." On the surface, the epileptoid is often highly moral and even religious. However, as soon as someone provokes them, they can instantly forget about their morality and cause significant harm or even kill. Later, when the emotions are discharged, the epileptoid regains composure and begins to reproach themselves, feeling strong guilt and remorse. They seek forgiveness, attempt to atone for their guilt, and promise that they will never behave that way again. And most importantly, they sincerely believe it. In reality, however, after some time passes and another irritating stimulus arises, there is a high probability that they will repeat what they did before. And the cycle repeats itself.

Once, one of our epileptoid patients came home, where he lived with his lover. As he later recounted, she kept provoking him for about three hours, and then he couldn't take it any-more and punched her in the jaw, causing significant physical injuries. The next morning, he took her to the hospital and then came to us for a consultation. He appeared crushed by feelings of guilt and shame, saying that he himself didn't understand how it happened, as if he fell into a trance where something else was controlling him. Similar situations occurred in his life from time to time, regardless of his attempts at volitional control, which is an extremely rare occurrence among individuals with an epileptoid profile. They most often follow their emotions and instincts, although they can be highly intellectual. This tendency often predisposes them to fights, promiscuous sexual relationships, alcohol and drug abuse.

If we are dealing not only with an epileptoid personality profile but with epilepsy as a disease, the influence of hypnosis and other practices altering the state of consciousness can trigger epileptoid seizures.

These seizures range from minor absences, where the patient seems to disconnect from consciousness while maintaining the same bodily position for several minutes, to a grand epileptoid seizure involving falling to the floor, rolling back the eyes, foaming at the mouth, and convulsions.

Therefore, some specialists do not recommend using hypno-sis with epilepsy patients due to the high likelihood of such an outcome.

During a lecture on psychotherapy where we conducted and demonstrated group hypnosis techniques, a student suffering from epilepsy, after emerging from trance, remained frozen with her eyes open and stayed in a similar state for a few minutes, barely breathing, before spontaneously returning to a normal waking state.

However, when she participated in holotropic breathwork group therapy, the epileptoid phenomenon of absence recurred. For a few minutes, it was as if she disconnected, stopped breathing, and then abruptly returned to her usual state of consciousness. She did not experience a major epileptic seizure.

Nevertheless, it is worth noting that she was highly hypnotizable. The hyperactive areas of the brain that could potentially trigger an epileptoid seizure during hypnosis can explosively discharge their tension.

On the one hand, this makes the trance healing for the patient, but on the other hand, it increases the likelihood of experiencing an epileptoid seizure.

Let us discuss how both individuals with epilepsy and those with an epileptoid profile have a very strong inner need to experience trance states and intuitively grasp such an opportunity as it provides them with psychoemotional relief.

It is precisely for this reason that epileptoid personalities often become hostages to alcohol, drugs, and various unpleasant emotional situations where excessive aggression is exhibited.

Speaking generally about the hypnotizability of epileptoid personalities, they are one of the most hypnotizable profiles. The trance emerges in the initial minutes of the hypnotic process, and the suggestee quickly reaches a high level of trance depth with numerous sensory and motor representations.

The influence of a typical relaxing and positive trance is not necessary for epileptoids. One trance session helps achieve high therapeutic indicators.

It is also worth noting that in trance, epileptoids tend to focus on experiencing bodily sensations, almost completely disregarding visual experiences. Therefore, the experience of visual hallucinations and illusions is nearly closed off to them.

At the same time, catalepsy of the hands and body, as well as hand levitation, can be relatively easily reproduced.

Among individuals with an epileptoid profile, we have discovered a very interesting common psychodynamic pattern. Almost all of them are "mother's children" and have limited or no significant connection with their father figure.

There is also another intriguing characteristic. They are not just "mother's children"; deep down in their souls, they fear their mothers. We often observed situations where the future epileptoid's mother did not want the child during pregnancy, either attempting to abort or contemplating it.

In our opinion, during the perinatal phase of their development, the child internalizes the aggression from the mother, and epileptoid seizures or simply epileptoid behavior serve as a form of catharsis, expressing the perinatal fear of the mother.

However, at this point, we merely propose this as a hypothesis that still requires repeated confirmation.

Key characteristics of the epileptoid type:

- Excitability
- Emotional uninhibition
- Aggressiveness, predominantly motor
- Lack of behavioral control during an affective outburst
- Feelings of guilt after the manifestation of an affect
- Hedonism
- Proneness to alcoholism and drug addiction
- Uninhibited sexuality
- Tendency to impulsively engage in socially disapproved actions
- Love for sports

Assessing the hypnotizability characteristics of the profile:

- Maximum level of hypnotizability
- Unlike the hysteroid profile, the external phenomenology of trance is relatively limited, but the internal manifestation of phenomena is highly extensive and diverse
- Both the induction of trance itself and the experiences within it have a strong psychogenic effect on the individual.

12

Schizophrenic Personality Profile

In our opinion, there is a fine line between the actual illness of schizophrenia and its personality accentuation. The ability for basic social adaptation serves as a key characteristic. If a person, due to specific symptoms indicating the presence of schizophrenia, can maintain socialization skills and derive pleasure from life, we refer to it as a schizophrenic accentuation. However, let us first describe the main forms of schizophrenia that can be observed in the clinical picture, and only then discuss the simple schizophrenic personality profile, which can differ significantly from a full-fledged disorder. In contemporary psychiatry, five primary subtypes of schizophrenia are most commonly recognized:

- **Paranoid schizophrenia**
- **Catatonic schizophrenia**
- **Hebephrenic schizophrenia**
- **Undifferentiated schizophrenia**
- **Residual schizophrenia**

Paranoid schizophrenia manifests through the emergence of various sensory illusions and hallucinations, most of which elicit a negative emotional response in the patient. Different personality distortions may arise, including absurd narcissism - megalomania, where a person begins to ascribe grandiose and peculiar identifications, such as Napoleon, Stalin, Director of the Universe, Chief Architect of Communism, Chairman of Planetary Forces, or even naming themselves after angels or demons, and so on. Patients may even create artificial credentials describing their "titles" and "accomplishments."

Naturally, absurd narcissism can be accompanied by hallucinatory processes and a strange worldview where the individual believes they are being pursued and tormented. In paranoid schizophrenia, the Kandinsky-Clérambault syndrome is manifested precisely in the hallucinatory delusion of persecution and influence on the subject. Such delusions of persecution can be conditionally divided into technical and magiphrenic types.

In the case of technical delusions, the patient may have fantasies that they are being irradiated with radiation, influenced by radio waves, laser beams, remotely hypnotized, implanted with "bugs" in their body, and so on. In magiphrenic delusions, the patient creates a picture of magical influence on themselves. They believe they are being bewitched, subjected to magical rituals, having enchanted objects thrown at them, having demons possess them, and so on. Naturally, the manifestation of symptoms is accompanied by vivid sensory experiences.

In the case of the reverse Kandinsky-Clérambault syndrome, the patient begins to believe that they themselves are the influencing subject. For example, they may think that they have the power to control the weather through their thoughts or that someone may die due to their bad mood. They believe

116

they can command and control a country, and so on.

Once, our former student brought her friend to us for a consultation. She had been diagnosed with paranoid schizophrenia two years ago, when she was 28 years old. The patient was actively taking antipsychotic medications, which caused behavioral and emotional suppression.

She recounted that when she was 28, she worked at a canteen in a local theater studio, and the symptoms began unexpectedly, appearing as strange paranoid fantasies telling her that the actors in the studio were gathering in the neighboring room to influence her through remote hypnosis, implant thoughts in her mind, and control her actions. Over the course of several weeks, the symptoms intensified, and then full-fledged kinesthetic hallucinations of certain entities emerged. These entities initially crawled on her skin and then began to crawl under her skin. One such spherical creature, twice the size of a tennis ball, settled beneath her right shoulder blade and occasionally moved, driving her to madness.

She sought help from psychiatrists, who prescribed neuroleptic therapy, which had little effect on her. Later, as she mentioned, she was given some experimental American medications, which also did not significantly reduce her symptom complex. Several months passed; orthodox medicine failed to help her, and she decided to seek unconventional healers, sorcerers, psychics, and exorcists. Sorcerers recited spells over her, all in vain. Psychics tried to cleanse her "aura," also with no success.

Interestingly, her unconventional treatment achieved some effect when she worked with Christian exorcists, who ritually performed prayers to expel demons from her. During each exorcism session, her symptoms took on new qualities. She would fall to the ground, crawl on all fours, hiss, grimace, and spit. After some time, the demon would "leave" her body, only to return again. Priests conducted this ritual several times, always with the same dramatic effect. There would be an outpouring of emotions, followed by a return to her previous state.

Our student, who was studying psychotherapy at our university, brought her to us to try hypnosis with her, hoping it might help. We knew that hypnotic practices with such patients rarely yielded any results. Nevertheless, we decided to give it a try for experimental purposes.

During our conversation and attempts to inquire about her childhood, she mostly responded in a monotonous and brief manner, clearly showing no attempts to remember anything. This could be due to strong resistance or the inability to engage in introspection due to neuroleptic intoxication. In essence, she was completely unresponsive to verbal analytic therapy, although she maintained relative social adequacy in communication. We attempted traditional Ericksonian hypnotic induction with her, and within five minutes, it became evident that it was ineffective for her. She displayed no signs of trance.

After some consideration, we decided to explore a hypnotic practice involving communication with different parts of her personality without a formal induction of trance. The hypnotherapist would simply address a specific part of the patient's personality and anticipate the patient's responses from that perspective. This practice resulted in a profound trance effect.

We administered a hypnotic intervention to the patient, directing our attention to the part of her personality located behind her right scapula. Following this intervention, the patient switched off, experiencing tremors throughout her body. Her chin dropped onto her chest, and her hair fell forward from her forehead. Then something unexpected happened. The patient fiercely hissed at us without opening her eyes, resembling a character from a horror movie. We attempted to engage in dialogue with the emerged part of her personality, but all we heard in response were hissing sounds. We then addressed the patient by her name, and she snapped back to herself. She had no awareness of what had transpired in the past couple of minutes. Questions regarding her conscious awareness yielded no results. We then turned our attention once again to the part of her personality located behind her right scapula and obtained a similar outcome as before. Thus, we transitioned her through different states multiple times, discovering that her consciousness resembled a television with two channels. On one channel, her own personality resided, while on the other, a hissing entity was present.

This particular case presented unique challenges for traditional hypnotic approaches. However, by employing a technique that involved communication with distinct parts of the patient's personality, we observed a profound transformation in her mental state. These findings contribute to the growing body of knowledge in the field of psychotherapy and highlight the potential benefits of alternative approaches in cases resistant to conventional methods.

It is important to note that further exploration and research are necessary to fully understand the mechanisms and efficacy of this type of hypnotherapeutic practice. Nonetheless, these preliminary results encourage further investigation into the utilization of personality-part-based communication techniques in the context of hypnosis, potentially opening new avenues for therapeutic interventions.

Thus, we can observe that classical clinical hypnosis may have no effect at all, but certain hypnotic practices can help to interact with the patient's consciousness to some extent.

Another one of our patients, also diagnosed with paranoid schizophrenia, was more talkative and even responsive to traditional forms of hypnotic induction. She came for therapy at the age of 35, with the onset of the schizophrenic process occurring at 30. Various hallucinations, perceptual illusions, deep and prolonged depression, and a loss of meaning in life began to manifest. Medication treatment with neuroleptics and antidepressants managed to alleviate most of the symptoms. However, the symptoms continued to interfere with her life and distort its quality. The patient was capable of engaging in analytical processes; during some consultations, she could reason reasonably, recall the past, and accept analytical interpretations. Occasionally, she would enter states where the quality of her communication significantly deteriorated. We noticed that to keep her in an adequate state, we simply needed to avoid certain topics in her life. Whenever we saw her slip into a negative state, we abruptly changed the conversation topic and observed how she subsequently stabilized. Her personality resembled a semi-ruined house. As long as her consciousness resided in one part, she remained completely adequate and stable. However, once her consciousness shifted to another part, she lost the adequacy of her perception of the world. During the analytical process, we discovered significant information about her personal history that had a pre-determining influence on the development of schizophrenia in her future. When she was seven years old, she was seduced by her twelve-year-old cousin, with whom she had an intimate relationship. According to her, during the course of therapy, her cousin was diagnosed with brain cancer. The development of the schizophrenic process in women who have been violated by a family member can be interpreted as a pattern that often appears in the personal histories of schizophrenic patients.

Naturally, we attempted several hypnosis sessions with her to assess the influence of trance on her consciousness and to explore the therapeutic resources within this technique. During the hypnotic induction process, contrary to our expectations, we discovered that the patient was quite hypnotizable, easily entering a hypnotic trance and experiencing a significant amount of sensory representations.

However, the most notable characteristic of her trance immersion was the constant presence of subtle demonic grimaces on her face. These grimaces would sometimes manifest as expressions of anger, pain, or suffering, alternating from one to another. We speculated that the appearance of these grimaces might lead to an escalation of negative emotional states, but it did not occur.

Upon emerging from the trance state, the patient reported feeling slightly more anxious and described the internal sensory representations as saturated with various negative emotional experiences. The imagery was predominantly black and white, with occasional bursts of red.

Over a period of three months, we predominantly employed analytical techniques while occasionally incorporating trance interventions during our work with the patient. Observable changes occurred, yet despite our efforts, we were unable to truly heal the wounded aspects of her personality. However, we discovered that we could teach her to voluntarily exit the symptomatic state.

In our opinion, the hypnotic technique neither caused harm nor provided significant benefits to the patient. Nevertheless, it was evident that the trance process could temporarily amplify the symptoms of the schizophrenic process.

Key characteristics of paranoid schizophrenia:

1. Hallucinations
2. Illusions
3. Autism
4. Impaired affective sphere
5. Associations based on secondary criteria
6. Ambivalence of thoughts and emotions
7. Problems in the volitional sphere
8. Apathy
9. Alogia (poverty of speech)
10. Anhedonia (inability to experience pleasure).

Evaluation of hypnotizability in a paranoid schizophrenic profile:

- The variations can be quite diverse. With the use of conventional techniques, the profile may not be hypnotizable at all. However, certain hypnosis techniques can induce peak hypnotic experiences.
- Trance enhances the propensity for fantasizing.
- In different cases, entering into a trance may be difficult, or specific forms of hypnotic induction may be necessary to achieve the desired result.
- Trance post-effects can have a negative bias and exacer-

bate negative symptoms.

When it comes to **catatonic schizophrenia**, the main manifestation of the illness is the prolonged, sometimes hours–long, immobility of the patient, known as catatonic stupor. The duration of this state can span hours, days, weeks, months, and even years.

At times, in catatonia, the patient's body is in a state of catalepsy, exhibiting a wax–like flexibility. The body can be positioned in any posture, and it will maintain fixation.

Sometimes catatonia can be negativistic, and attempts to change the patient's posture are met with strong resistance.

There is also a deeper form of catatonia called tetany, where attempts to alter the patient's position can result in such intense muscular tension that it may even cause internal organ injuries.

Sometimes catatonia can be intermittent, where, for example, a patient remains in stupor for several weeks and then unexpectedly transitions into a state of catatonic excitement. They may perform certain actions, often aggressive ones, and then return to the catatonic state. In one such case, a patient remained in a stupor for several weeks. While under the observation of doctors in a clinic, he suddenly emerged from the catatonic state, grabbed a metal bowl, and threw it at a passing orderly. The orderly managed to dodge, remaining unharmed. The doctor asked him to explain his actions some time later, to which he replied that while he was in the stupor, an inner voice repeated the phrase "move and you'll die, move and you'll die" to him. At one point, the voice told him, "if you kill the orderly with the bowl, you'll be saved; now throw it." After the patient missed, the voice began repeating that he was now doomed. In this case, we can observe that the internal vocal interpretation influences the behavior of the patient and their states.

There are three forms of catatonic excitement that can be distinguished:

Gradual speech and motor excitement are accompanied by speech emphasis and sometimes echolalia, heightened mood, and exaltation. Unprovoked laughter may occur. Impulsive actions are possible, but without disturbance of consciousness.

Acute and rapid speech and motor excitement. Behavior includes echolalia, echopraxia, and perseveration. Actions are aggressive and chaotic. Self-harm is possible.

Mute excitement. Agitation, chaotic and purposeless actions, self-inflicted harm, and harm to others.

Catatonia can also manifest through the following symptoms:

1. Mutism (silence)
2. Active or passive negativism
3. Echolalia (repeating the words of others)
4. Echopraxia (repeating the actions and movements of others)
5. Pillow sign
6. Ivan Pavlov's sign (understanding and reacting only to a quiet voice)
7. Jactitations (voluntary stereotypical rocking of the body and head)

We can hypothesize that the phrases that govern the behavior of schizophrenic individuals are implanted in their minds during childhood by someone close to them, most often their father or mother, during intensely stressful situations where the child may have felt fear and pain.

Unfortunately, obtaining detailed information about the childhood experiences of patients with such symptoms is not easy. It is often nearly impossible, so we are left with assumptions and hypotheses, but not unfounded ones.

Based on what we have observed in some patients, if the childhood experience involved intense fear and pain coupled with someone's implantation of commands like "do something" or "don't do something," this implantation may transform into a strong, uncontrollable symptom in adulthood.

For example, a woman with the rather unusual symptom of selective abulia (lack of will) sought the help of a psychotherapist. She couldn't say no to anyone, even in various contexts of her life. For instance, a stranger could approach her on the street and tell her to "follow me," and she would comply.

This selective abulia had a psychoanalytic justification. When the patient was 5 years old, she was playing in the kitchen while her mother was cooking on the stove. She somehow upset her mother, who instructed her to sit on a chair. The daughter shouted, "No, I don't want to." In response, her mother slammed her hand on the table, where there was a cup of boiling water, causing it to spill onto the child, and she yelled, "Never say no to me!"

This had a profound suggestive impact on the daughter. In fact, after that incident, she couldn't say no to anyone. Such was the power of suggestion. Indeed, intense pain and fear can open the subconscious to suggestion, and it becomes extremely difficult to free oneself from the influence of that suggestion.

However, more often, similar phrases from childhood form

various phobias, obsessions, and compulsions. But we will hypothesize that similar events from personal childhood experiences can also account for the imperative phrases described above in the mind of a catatonic schizophrenic. However, this is a psychoanalytic interpretation.

When considering other factors, the causes of catatonia can be other mental disorders or physical illnesses. For example, in ICD-11, there are categories such as "catatonia associated with other mental disorders," "catatonia induced by psychoactive substances, including medications," and "secondary catatonic syndrome." Today, the belief is growing that catatonia is more often a consequence of affective disorders than schizophrenia. In any case, this question remains open.

The development of catatonic stupor or excitement can be influenced by:

Mental disorders:

- Affective disorders
- Post-traumatic stress disorder (PTSD)
- Postpartum mental disorders
- Developmental disorders in children

Neurological symptoms:

- History of cranial-brain trauma
- Brain tumor
- Stroke

Use of certain medications and drugs:

- Antipsychotics (malignant neuroleptic syndrome)
- Anticonvulsants
- Corticosteroids
- Cocaine, phencyclidine, opioids

As we can see, there are many different causes, and catatonic syndrome can occur in various conditions, not limited to schizophrenia spectrum disorders. However, for now, we will continue to associate catatonia specifically with the spectrum of schizophrenic mental disorders.

Bringing a person out of a catatonic stupor is often very challenging. However, some psychiatrists and psychotherapists may occasionally employ unconventional behavioral patterns to achieve the desired effect.

For example, Frank Farrelly used extremely extreme forms of behavior with his patients. He would start plucking hair from the legs of a patient who was stuck in a catatonic stupor, gradually moving upward from the knee toward the groin. He would say to the patient, "I will continue doing this higher and higher!" Eventually, the patient would emerge from the stupor and slap Frank. This is not a treatment method, but this example illustrates that certain behavioral maneuvers can lead a patient out of a catatonic stupor.

Unfortunately, we have not found any indications in the literature regarding any experiments with hypnotic suggestion in patients suffering from catatonia. However, we can make the assumption that, in some cases, hypnotic influence may have therapeutic potential.

Evaluation of hypnability in schizophrenic catatonic profiles:

· Undifferentiated

In the **hebephrenic subtype of schizophrenia**, the symptom progression follows the following characteristics. The behavior exhibits pronounced features such as:

· Childishness.
· Foolishness.
· Elevated mood.
· Affected mannerisms.
· Delusional ideas.
· Aggressive actions.
· Unfounded behaviors.
· Bizarre and indecent behavior.
· Giggling.
· Grimaces.
· Pranks.
· Hallucinations may be present.

This subtype of schizophrenia was first identified by Evald Hecker in his medical practice in 1878. He described this disorder as follows: "The onset during the period of sexual maturity... rapid transition into a state of mental weakness and a specific form of terminal stupidity, the signs of which could be recognized in the early stages of the illness."

The diagnosis of hebephrenic schizophrenia is most commonly made during adolescence and early adulthood (14–18 years). Without partial drug remission, almost all forms of verbal therapy are impractical.

Similar to catatonic schizophrenia, we have not found any experimental data on the use of hypnotic suggestion in patients with this symptom.

Evaluation of hypnability in an undifferentiated schizophrenic profile:

· Undifferentiated

In **undifferentiated schizophrenia**, we observe a combination of symptoms from various types of schizophrenia, making it impossible to establish a clear diagnosis.

Generalized schizophrenia manifests in a specific form of altered social behavior, sometimes with superficial relative normalcy in the patient. Let's describe the key features of the psychological processes and behavioral reactions associated with this type of mental disorder.

The individual almost completely loses their circle of familiar contacts and ceases to take care of themselves. They may go unwashed for weeks or months and not wash their clothes, resulting in a noticeable, unpleasant odor. They lose employment and educational pursuits, as well as motivation towards them.

Intellectual activities are often minimized to reading tabloids or shallow fiction literature. They may spend hours watching movies or playing online games. They develop their own life philosophy and can talk extensively about it. To an outsider, they may appear to possess a philosophical mindset. However, upon closer examination of their speech, it becomes evident that it is not a philosophical text but rather an absurd combination of meanings.

Apathy sets in, leading to significant difficulties in setting goals and following through with them. On one day, they can genuinely express to others their intention to change their life, return to university, or find employment, only to completely forget their grand speeches the next day and continue playing their online game. Their emotional life becomes reduced.

Abstract terms and words abound in their thinking and speech. Their sexual life is often either absent or dominated by autoeroticism. They encounter significant challenges in form- ing intimate sexual relationships, and if such relationships occur, they tend to end quickly. They are less likely to smoke, consume alcohol, or use drugs, indicating a potentially elevated level of dopamine and GABA neurotransmitter secretion. They may sometimes exhibit a tendency toward overeating.

They dislike sports and any form of intense physical activity, leading to significant muscle atrophy. This factor indicates an extremely low level of norepinephrine neurotransmitter in the brain. They often do not experience hallucinations, unlike patients with other types of schizophrenia. It is precisely because of this that cases are common where the patient's behavior is attributed by their loved ones to their personality, laziness, or other social factors.

Let's describe one case of observing such a patient and comment on their ability to interact with trance states.

A 25-year-old young man enrolled in a university where we taught the subject of psychotherapy. Initially, he showed an interest in studying and joined the psychotherapeutic group we led. He mentioned that this was already his third university enrollment. He had been expelled from previous ones due to non-attendance.

After enrolling in previous universities, he would gradually lose interest in education and stop attending classes. He followed the following unconscious behavioral pattern. Initially, he would make friends at the university and attend classes, but after six months or longer, something would switch within him. He would stay at home, watching anime for up to ten hours a day, playing online games, and hardly ever leaving the house. His spatial movement was primarily limited to the kitchen, bathroom, and toilet. He remained unemployed during this time.

After six months of this routine, he would snap out of it. He would return to the university, only to find out that he had been expelled. A similar pattern was repeated at another university with almost identical timeframes. While studying at the third university, he assured us that he would now focus on his education and complete it. In our opinion, thanks to his participation in the therapy group, his next crisis occurred only after a year and a half of studying.

He started dating a girl from another group, but she broke up with him. Then, a few months later, around New Year's, after arguing with his father, she came to his house, and they entered into a romantic relationship. They broke up after a month, and after that, he experienced a significant decline in mood and motivation in his studies. He continued attending therapy groups for some time but stopped taking care of himself, not bathing, emitting a strong odor that concerned other group members, and engaging in absurd philosophical conversations.

He soon stopped attending the group and resumed his familiar pathological routine, where he stayed at home, ate, and watched anime. He remained in this state until the end of the academic year at the university. When invited to return to the university, he usually responded that he would return soon but never showed up. After completing the academic year, he was expelled.

After that, his brother came to us and informed us that he was staying at home. The brother also mentioned that he said a strange phrase after being expelled: "Now I'll finally live!" When asked what he meant, he replied, "Now no one will interrupt me from watching anime." What happened to him afterward is unknown to us.

In all of his six-month-long home "hibernations," he exhibited almost the entire spectrum of symptoms characteristic of general schizophrenia. An interesting feature of these symptoms was that they would occur, on average, twice a year, lasting for about six months each time. We were unable to determine the cause of such a cyclic reproduction of symptoms.

During his participation in therapy and educational groups, we conducted numerous hypnotherapy sessions with him. In all sessions, he demonstrated himself as an excellent hypnotic suggestible subject. He most frequently reached medium and deep levels of trance, experiencing a significant number of sensations and meanings. However, he encountered difficulties manifesting trance phenomena. We were unable to induce catalepsy or levitation. Similar problems arose when attempting to reproduce other phenomena. Although the overall trance state could be quite deep, we have yet to find a comprehensive explanation for this phenomenon. Nonetheless, we speculate that the cyclic social demotivation experienced by the patient is naturally associated with a decrease in norepinephrine levels and an increase in dopamine levels in the brain. Additionally, we hypothesize that excessive dopamine secretion in certain areas of the brain in patients with general schizophrenia may block the ability to reproduce hypnotic phenomena. In our opinion, social activity and hypnotic activity may share a similar nature in our brain. In a typical individual, the reproduction of social actions and trance phenomena is reinforced by increased dopamine levels. In patients with general schizophrenia, this chemical motivational mechanism is disrupted both in the social sphere and during the hypnotherapy process.

Key characteristics of the general schizophrenic type:

1. Alogia: poverty of speech or lack of verbal fluency.
2. Abulia: decreased motivation and inability to initiate or persist in goal-directed activities.
3. Apathy: lack of interest, enthusiasm, or emotional responsiveness.
4. Anhedonia: inability to experience pleasure or derive enjoyment from previously enjoyable activities.
5. Autism: social withdrawal and limited engagement in social interactions.
6. Problems with emotional expression: difficulties in expressing emotions or displaying appropriate emotional responses.
7. Associations based on secondary cues: making connections or associations between unrelated things based on superficial similarities.
8. Ambivalence of thoughts and emotions: conflicting thoughts, feelings, or motivations.
9. Disheveled appearance: neglect of personal hygiene or grooming.
10. Absence or near absence of sexual life.
11. Difficulties in forming and maintaining friendships.
12. Absence of visual, auditory, and kinesthetic hallucinations

and illusions.
13. Superficial impression of personal peculiarity or eccentricity.
14. Pseudophilosophizing: engaging in abstract or philosophical discussions with little coherence or depth.

Assessment of hypnotizability in the general schizophrenic profile:

1. Moderate to strong hypnotizability with possible unusual emotional affective responses.
2. Hypnosis may enhance the inclination for fantasizing.
3. Hypnosis may exhibit a tendency towards oneiric (dream-like) experiences or anxiety-phobic tendencies.

13

Manic-Depressive Personality Profile

Patients with manic-depressive psychosis (or bipolar affective disorder, BAR) experience cyclical episodes of intense mood elevation (mania) and mood depression, accompanied by various associated psycho-emotional and behavioral reactions. Different combinations of these states are possible, and the patient exhibits distinctly different symptoms during the two main phases of the illness.

In the manic phase, the following symptoms accompany the individual:

- Elevated mood
- Motor agitation
- Ideational and mental excitement
- Spiritual uplift
- Rapid and verbose speech
- Increased sexual drive
- Increased appetite
- Aggressive behavior
- Reduced need for sleep

- Possible emergence of grandiose delusions
- Almost complete absence of guilt or shame for actions

In the depressive phase, the following symptoms accompany the individual:

- Low mood
- Motor retardation
- Spiritual decline
- Slowed speech
- Decreased sexual drive
- Decreased appetite
- Increased need for sleep
- Feelings of worthlessness
- Suicidal impulses may occur
- Prolonged immobility
- Persistent self-condemnation and moral self-torment
- Apathy (problems with volition)
- Loss of social interest

As we can see here, the symptoms of the two stages have diametrically opposite qualities. The intensity of their manifestation can vary greatly. The course of Bipolar Affective Disorder (BAD) can occur in the following forms:

1. Periodic mania (alternating only between mania and a neutral state)
2. Periodic depression (alternating only between depression and a neutral state)
3. Regularly alternating type (mania followed by depression and depression followed by mania)

4. Irregularly alternating type (a single phase may repeat multiple times, with mania followed by mania or depression followed by depression)
5. Circular type (there is no intermission when the phases alternate regularly)

If we consider Bipolar Affective Disorder (BAD) at the level of personality accent, we will notice that the alternation of mild manias and depressions will be sublimated by the social context. In other words, both phases can be socially productive for the individual.

However, when we examine borderline and psychotic BAD, we observe significant distortions in behavior within the social context, making the individual socially maladaptive.

It is worth noting that the manic phase itself is not always malignant. Sometimes, patients genuinely enjoy life during this period. The price is paid when transitioning into the depressive phase. Let's provide an example based on our observation of a patient with a mild form of BAD.

A 28-year-old woman experiences one manic and one depressive phase once a year. Each phase lasts for 3−4 months. The manic phase occurs at the end of spring, while the depressive phase occurs at the end of autumn. During the manic phase, she becomes highly energetic, actively engages in her activities, and organizes or develops her business relationships. She starts earning significantly more money. Her libido increases, resulting in a mild fear of infidelity towards her spouse, as she knows from experience that she is capable of it in such a state. She sleeps little and experiences joy in almost any activity. When we interacted with her during this phase, she left an impression of a warm, communicative, and optimistic person. She talks a lot and constantly makes jokes. People enjoy being around her. However, when the depressive phase sets in, she spends days sitting at home, unable to go to work, lying in bed. Thoughts fill her mind that she is a failure, that nothing good will happen in her life anymore, and that she won't be able to escape this state. She sleeps a lot and has little desire for sex. Closer to spring, this phase starts to fade, and she enters a neutral interphase. This yearly cyclic pattern has been repeating for many years, and the patient has become accustomed to it. Her main complaint is the loss of almost all social communication during the depressive phase, which leads to a decline in her business and relationships. During the depressive phase, she stops attending psychotherapy sessions.

For hypnotherapy, the most favorable time is the interphase, where patients, according to our observations, demonstrate a weak or moderate level of hypnotizability. They exhibit only certain hypnotic phenomena such as hand catalepsy, hand levitation, and motor analog signaling. In the manic and depressive phases, patients either do not enter a trance state at all or have a low level of hypnotizability.

During our work with patients suffering from Bipolar Affective Disorder (BAD), we discovered a common element in their birth history. Almost all patients with BAD were born with significant difficulties and various physical traumas. One had a clavicle fracture, another had a thigh injury, a third had forceps extraction, and so on. From this, we can hypothesize that a predisposition to manic-depressive-type disorders may arise precisely due to physical trauma during the birthing process. And cycloid affective processes that appear later in life can be seen as a certain form of abreaction and catharsis (psycho-emotional reaction) to the experienced shock and pain.

Assessment of the hypnotizability profile:

In this case, it makes sense to differentiate the effects of trance induction during the manic and depressive phases.

Manic phase:

- Moderate level of hypnotizability
- Exclusively positive orientation of trance content
- Always complete satisfaction with the trance experience
- Always satisfied with short-term psychotherapeutic dynamics

Depressive phase:

- Low or moderate level of hypnotizability
- More often, a negative orientation of trance process content
- Dissatisfaction with the trance experience

14

Psychopathological Personality Accents

Schizoid Accent	Psychopathic Accent	Schizophrenic Accent
Hysteroid Accent		Paranoid Accent
Manic-Depressive Accent	Obsessive-Compulsive Accent	Epileptoid Accent

The table displays the polarization of personality accents, namely:

Hysteroid Accent - Paranoid Accent

This pair is undoubtedly the true opposite on almost all psychological and physiological criteria. Hysteroids are highly hypnotizable, while paranoids are almost non-hypnotizable.

Psychopathic Accent - Obsessive-Compulsive Accent

Psychopaths are incapable of experiencing feelings of guilt and shame, whereas individuals with obsessive-compulsive accent are predominantly driven by these emotions.

Schizoid Accent - Epileptoid Accent

Schizoids are emotionally cold, withdrawn, unemotional, head-driven, rationalistic, and do not enjoy physical movement. They are not prone to alcoholism or drug addiction. Epileptoids are emotionally passionate, live through bodily sensations, are irrational, and enjoy movement. They are prone to alcoholism and drug addiction.

Schizophrenic Accent - Manic-Depressive Accent

During the manifestation of schizophrenia symptoms, we encounter a constant internal unresolved conflict and ambivalence of three types:

1. **Emotional**: simultaneous positive and negative feelings toward a person, object, or event.
2. **Volitional**: endless oscillations between opposing decisions. Inability to make a choice.
3. **Intellectual**: operating with mutually exclusive ideas and thoughts. In the manic-depressive accent, internal ambivalence seems to be divided into different temporal segments and experienced sequentially, rather than simultaneously.

In the MD accent, internal ambivalence is emphasized, as if it is divided into different time periods and is not translated simultaneously but sequentially.

By using this model for patient profiling based on the eight basic psychopathological types, we have found that with a high level of probability, we can effectively determine their ability to enter a trance state, the effectiveness of trance work, and the expected capacity to reproduce various trance phenomena.

15

Hypnotic Phenomena

There are a considerable number of perception and conscious-ness phenomena that can be created through hypnotic sugges-tion and trance work. Some of them naturally arise during the process of trance immersion, while others need to be specifically induced through trance induction. Certain phe-nomena can be adapted for psychotherapeutic purposes, while others are solely intended to demonstrate the capabilities of the hypnotic process. Let us explore their variety.

Eyelid catalepsy
During trance induction, a person's eyelids close and cannot be raised voluntarily. This phenomenon was observed by the mesmerist Lafontaine and the creator of the term "hypnosis," John Braid.

Eyelid lowering
Upon a hypnotic command, a person's eyelids lower. In the vast majority of cases, eyelid lowering occurs naturally and is perceived as the beginning of a hypnotic state. However, open

eyes are not an indication of the absence of a hypnotic trance. Typically, the hypnotic state is perceived almost exclusively as an externally oriented process. But this is one of the misconceptions about the hypnotic process. In many cases, trance can be maintained with open eyes and even with full body mobility. However, for the purpose of the psychotherapeutic process, transitioning the trance to an externally oriented state is often simply unnecessary.

Eyelid raising
Upon a hypnotic command, the eyelids are raised while maintaining the hypnotic state. In this case, a similar suggestion can be used, for example: "Now I will snap my fingers, and after that, your eyes will open while the depth of the trance state remains." Subsequently, additional suggestions can be given to regain control over speech function and initiate a dialogue with the suggestee.

Eyelid tremor
This is a spontaneously occurring phenomenon in which the eyelids begin to vibrate or tremble. It often occurs when the eyes roll upwards towards the brow and the head is tilted backward.

Catalepsy of the limbs and head
This is a spontaneously occurring or intentionally created phenomenon of wax-like flexibility. When a certain body part is placed in a new position, it remains independently held for an extended period of time.

Levitation of the hands

This is a spontaneously occurring or intentionally created phenomenon of unconscious lifting and movement of the hands in space. Rarely, during the induction of trance in hysterical patients, spontaneous raising of the hands into the air, sometimes accompanied by various movements, can be observed. In other cases, specific suggestions are required to activate this phenomenon.

Floppy hand syndrome

This phenomenon spontaneously occurs during hypnotic induction. The person loses voluntary control over hand movements. Regardless of the new position given by the hypnotist, the hands consistently fall downward. Suggestion that the hands maintain a fixed position often does not work. This phenomenon can be artificially recreated in individuals who can reproduce hand catalepsy. With the command "your hand becomes floppy, relaxed, and heavy," it drops down onto the knees. According to our observations, individuals who spontaneously reproduce this phenomenon can maintain it after numerous attempts. We have seen a patient who, despite having a relative ability to enter a hypnotic trance, continued to reproduce this phenomenon throughout a year of hypnotherapy. However, at one point, her hand became stuck in a cataleptic state.

Floppy body syndrome

This spontaneously occurs in some hysterically accentuated individuals. After entering a state of hypnotic trance, the entire body deeply relaxes, causing the person to completely lose conscious and unconscious muscle tone. If not supported, the person simply falls in any direction. In this case, no commands indicating the preservation of muscle tone are effective. This phenomenon can be artificially reproduced in individuals who are not prone to floppy body syndrome through specific hypnotic commands. For example: "Your body becomes soft and pliable, you lose all control over it."

Catalepsy of the entire body

A favorite old technique of European psychiatrists, regularly demonstrated in clinics with hysteric women. During hypnotization, either spontaneously or through appropriate suggestion, the body acquires wax-like flexibility. Regardless of the position it is placed in, it remains fixed. By securing the body in an upright position, the hypnotist, with the assistance of an accomplice, can place the subject between the backs of chairs (the upper part of the back on one chair and the lower part of the calves on another), creating a small cataleptic bridge. Another version of the cataleptic bridge is possible when the subject is held by the arms and lifted above their heads (one person holds the shoulders, while another holds the legs). In this case, we observe a larger cataleptic bridge.

Another variation is the acrobatic bridge

In this case, after inducing catalepsy of the entire body, the hypnotist, from a standing position, slowly begins to arch the subject's body backward, gradually placing their hands on the floor. This phenomenon can only be achieved if there is sufficient flexibility in the thoracic spine.

Hypnotic anesthesia

The phenomenon of depriving a specific area of the body of general sensitivity. Often reproduced together with the phenomenon of analgesia, which refers to the absence of pain sensitivity in a specific area of the body. Formally, anesthesia can be considered a negative kinesthetic hallucination.

Both anesthesia and analgesia usually do not occur spontaneously in a trance state but are induced through appropriate suggestions. In a training format, the technique of analgesia can be tested through an exercise involving the application of pressure to a painful point located at the base of the thumb and index finger. Initially, pressure is applied to the point, and the level of pain sensitivity is noted.

Then, a hypnotic exercise called the "Iron Glove" is performed in an externally oriented trance format. During one of the seminars, French psychiatrist Claude Viro demonstrated the following execution of this exercise. After the pain sensitivity test on the hand is conducted without formally inducing a trance, the hypnotist begins to speak, asking the subject to imagine wrapping their hand with chain mail, like a bandage, and to imagine, hear, and feel this sensation. Then, the suggestion is given to imagine placing a large steel glove over the chain mail on the hand, which will provide protection. This visualization is maintained for 2–3 minutes.

After the visualization is completed, the hypnotist attempts to apply pressure to the painful point on the hand again. Feedback is obtained from the subject regarding the difference in pain sensitivity between the first and second application of pressure. Based on our observations, in the majority of cases, the intensity of the pain sensations decreases by 4–5 times.

Another interesting exercise we witnessed was performed by a female physician in a French clinic. She aimed to alleviate the pain in the arm of a young girl in order to take some tests without discomfort. She took a regular marker in her hand, showed it to the girl, and told her that it was a magic marker that could relieve pain when it touches the body. She then slowly approached the girl's arm with the marker, lightly touched it, and began making spiral massaging movements along the forearm using the marker's cap. After just a minute of such a procedure, the girl lost both general and specific pain sensitivity in her arm.

Once the tests were taken, the physician ran the marker cap backward along the forearm, explaining that the sensitivity was returning to the arm. At first, it may seem like magic, but in reality, this exercise is quite simple to replicate and does not even require prior hypnotic induction. The phenomenon is solely created by focusing attention on the object and establishing suggestive ideas about its function and purpose.

A completely different form of analgesia is applied during surgical procedures. According to available information, full hypnotic analgesia was first performed by an English physician in India during the Indian Company in the late 19th century. The records indicate that amputation surgery was performed under hypnosis for the purpose of pain control. Since then, military physicians have started using hypnosis in dentistry. More and more evidence was emerging, indicating that hypnosis could be an effective analgesic agent.

Currently, hypnotic anesthesia is used during surgical operations in numerous European and American clinics. For example, in French clinics, hypnotic anesthesia is employed during surgeries performed under local anesthesia. In such cases, hypnotic anesthesia serves as a substitute for general anesthesia.

Before the start of the surgery, the hypnotherapist begins by directing the patient's attention to various external objects. The patient undergoes 4-5 attention fixations. Then the patient is asked to close their eyes and imagine themselves in a specific trance motif, such as being on a seaside. After that, for ten minutes, the hypnotherapist, in a soft and slow voice, guides the patient on a journey through the trance motif, focusing their attention on visual, auditory, and kinesthetic sensations that the patient can experience during the hypnosis session. For example: "And you can see the yellow sand and the blue sea... And you can hear the sound of the wind and the cry of seagulls... And feel the wind blowing through your hair...". Such phrases are repeated cyclically many times.

When the patient has been in the trance for more than ten minutes, the surgeons begin the surgical intervention. During the procedure, the hypnotherapist remains beside the patient and continues to accompany them with their voice through the trance motif. This continues until the end of the surgery. The gradual transition out of trance begins when the operation is completed and the sutures are applied.

Naturally, the patient has a choice before the surgery: either to undergo it with full medication anesthesia or to choose local and hypnotherapeutic anesthesia. In the case of choosing the latter option, there is always the possibility, if the hypnotic form of anesthesia does not work sufficiently well, of switching the patient to full medication anesthesia. However, in the vast majority of cases, this is not necessary. Hypnotic anesthesia is used with people of various age groups: children, adults, and elderly individuals. According to observations by French medical professionals, postoperative recovery is faster for individuals who choose hypnotic pain management. There has also been an increase in self-confidence among individuals who undergo hypnotic anesthesia.

During the training format for the implementation of the technique of hypnotherapeutic anesthesia and analgesia, it is possible to use small needles to puncture the skin on the hands or forearms. The depth of the puncture is superficial, just enough for the needle to pass through the epidermis. In addition to the above-mentioned methods of creating hypnotic pain management, direct suggestion can also be employed. For example: "Your hand ceases to feel pain, the sensitivity in it decreases to a minimum, and it is protected from any external interference." Working with various metaphors is also possible, for instance: "You are standing on the shore of a frozen lake, piercing a hole in the ice and inserting your hand into it, feeling a strong coldness in your hand spreading up to your shoulder. Your hand freezes and is covered with a layer of ice; you cannot feel anything except the coldness in it." This is an example of a metaphor that can be vividly developed during trance, adding more descriptive elements to depict sensations of different qualities.

Usually, when suggestion or metaphor (or both) are successfully activated in trance, a person does not feel any pain during the needle puncture. Sometimes the sensation is simply very weak and superficial.

Bleeding cessation

Hypnotic techniques can be used to attempt to stop minor bleeding. An interesting example of an experiment with blood cessation during gum surgery was shared by Claude Viro in a seminar. In one instance, during gum surgery where hypoanalgesia was applied, the patient experienced severe bleeding that the doctor could not stop. Seizing the oppor-

tunity, the hypnotherapist decided to try to stop the bleeding using hypnosis. He suggested to the patient that they
were in front of a lever that controlled the intensity of the
bleeding, and they could touch it to adjust its settings. Then
he suggested that, in the patient's imagination, they visually
changed the lever, reducing its intensity to a minimum. Within
a minute, the bleeding actually ceased to flow intensively.
As an experimental continuation, he then suggested to the
patient that they reverse the direction of the lever. The blood
started flowing intensely again. Finally, he suggested the
patient return the setting to the minimum, and once again, the
suggestion worked. In this case, we can see an example of using
functional visual metaphors to interact with and potentially
alter not only a person's state but also the course of certain
physiological processes.

A similar example of working with functional visual metaphors
can be found in the works of American hypnotherapist Leslie
LeCron, who was active in the 1950s and 1970s. Here's the
story of a case he encountered. Once, a patient came to LeCron
for a session and complained about a toothache, mentioning
that after the psychotherapy session, they would have to visit a
dentist to have it extracted. LeCron suggested using hypnosis
to anesthetize the toothache, and the patient agreed. LeCron
induced a hypnotic state and suggested that the patient was in
a "consciousness control room," instructing them to find the
button to turn off the toothache on the control panel. He then
asked the patient to mentally press the button. Afterwards, he
brought the patient out of a trance. Remarkably, the pain was
indeed turned off. Subsequently, the patient went to the dentist.
When they returned for the next session with LeCron, they

reported that the entire dental procedure had been surprisingly painless, which amazed both the patient and the dentist.

Regarding functional visual panels, it's worth noting that Richard Bandler extensively applied them in his psychother-apeutic method called DHE (Design Human Engineering), which he developed in the mid-1980s. Bandler significantly expanded the functional application of these panels and created a range of techniques that allow for the alteration of numerous states, whether in collaboration with a psychotherapist or independently. Similar DHE techniques will be presented in the practical section of the book.

Hypnotic hyperesthesia

By hypnotic hyperesthesia, we understand the emergence of various sensations in the body that are not typical in the ordinary waking state of consciousness. For example, this may involve the experience of warmth or coldness, heaviness or lightness, vibrations, or sensations of movement within the body, and so on. This phenomenon can occur naturally during trance induction or can be artificially induced through suggestion.

Hypnotic Amnesia

This phenomenon refers to the partial or complete loss of the ability to remember a specific period of time in a patient. Dur-ing hypnotic suggestion, amnesia can occur spontaneously or be induced. In almost all cases, spontaneous amnesia is formed only during the period of hypnotic induction. For example, a patient may remember the beginning of the hypnosis session and the moment of coming out of it, but forget what exactly happened during the trance induction. This phenomenon is quite commonly observed and often appears during the induction of deep levels of hypnotic trance. Hypnotic amnesia can also be suggested for the patient. We provided a similar example in the section of the book dedicated to the hysteric profile of personality. In our opinion, this profile is almost ideal for reproducing this phenomenon. With representatives of other profiles, even highly hypnotizable ones, reproducing this phenomenon is not often successful, or it creates an *illusion of amnesia*—a phenomenon similar to amnesia that gives the feeling that the memory is still there but there is no desire to recall it at the moment.

Richard Bandler once shared a story about successfully suggesting to a patient during a hypnosis session that he had forgotten he ever smoked. The patient spent several days wondering why his smoking acquaintances kept offering him cigarettes. Eventually, the amnesia naturally disappeared. Inspired by this, we decided to conduct a similar experiment but with a slight variation. In one hypnosis laboratory, we took one of our students with a hysteric profile of personality who despised nicotine and cringed at the smell of cigarette smoke. We induced her into a state of deep hypnotic trance and suggested to her that she had been smoking cigarettes for a long time and enjoyed it. Then we brought her out of trance, left the room with her, and offered her a cigarette. She calmly took it and happily lit it. We then re-induced her into trance, removed the previous suggestion, and brought her back to the waking state, where she again reacted very negatively to nicotine. Formally, this could be called *mnesic illusion*, a phenomenon where a person becomes convinced that something occurred in the experience that did not actually happen.

We performed another experiment with the same student to create selective amnesia. We suggested to her that she forget how to use the Ukrainian language and that her native language be English. It is worth noting that she knew English at a basic level. After coming out of trance, she did not understand Russian words addressed to her and responded in English phrases. At our request, she took out her passport from her bag. After she failed to read anything from it, she exclaimed, "Oh my God, I can't read this text!" Then we re-induced her into a trance and canceled the previous suggestions. Such experiments vividly demonstrate the ability of our consciousness to recreate various hypnotic phenomena associated with memory functioning.

Hypnotic Recall

This trance phenomenon allows the resurfacing of forgotten fragments in memory through hypnotic suggestion. It can occur spontaneously or through appropriate suggestion. Spontaneous hypnotic recall may manifest during hypnosis as the recollection of forgotten parts of one's personal history. These parts of personal history are often emotionally charged and require psychotherapeutic processing. These memories can emerge as full-fledged internal films and images, where the person immediately recognizes which memory they are dealing with and to which time period it belongs.

Cathartic Remembrance

Sometimes, cathartic remembrance may occur, which involves a strong emotional abreaction such as laughter, tears, vomiting, and so on. For example, during a hypnotic regression into early childhood, our patient began to cry while remaining in a hypnotic trance. When we brought her out of the trance state and asked what she specifically remembered from her childhood, she replied that in her recollection, she became a six-year-old girl again, and her mother wanted to take her to school, but she didn't want to go and started crying. In this case, during the hypnotic induction, we did not provide any suggestions for the patient to recall a specific memory. What manifested was a spontaneous expression of cathartic hyper-mnesia. Sometimes, the intense expression of emotions during trance induction can occur without consciously recognizing the exact memory fragment from which it arises. However, we most often observed such phenomena when working with the holotropic breathwork technique, where individuals can laugh, cry, and scream without fully realizing the source of the emotional abreaction.

An interesting example of unconscious strong emotional abreaction was witnessed during one of Bert Hellinger's sem-inars. Instead of using his systemic constellation method with a patient, he created a hypnotic regression using physical perinatal anchoring. He embraced the patient in a circle with his arms and then asked her to start freeing herself from his therapeutic embrace, which triggered her experience of reliving her birth. The patient spent about 15 minutes going through the "birth paths" out of Bert's embrace and then fell to the ground. Afterwards, the participants helped her lie down on chairs next to Bert, resting her head on his lap. She re-mained there for another 20 minutes. Throughout this process, Hellinger described the metaphor of a journey up the staircase of life, where each step symbolized a year of the patient's life. Ascending the stairs recreated the phenomenon of hypnotic progression in her consciousness. Hellinger carefully observed the patient's nonverbal reactions to each year of her life, and if he noticed that a particular emotion began to surface, he would pause for a while. In some childhood years, the patient exhibited body tremors and tears. Around the third or fourth year, she started vomiting. Hellinger commented that she had experienced intense emotional struggles that year. From the age of 5–6 and into adulthood, no significant negative experiences were observed.

Another example from our practice involved a patient who had attempted suicide by hanging four years prior to seeking psychotherapy, resulting in partial retrograde amnesia for the last two years of her life. We attempted to help her retrieve the forgotten fragments using hypnotic work. In the hypnotic session, we used an externally oriented trance. We placed pieces of paper on the floor in a line, symbolizing the timeline, and the paper scraps represented fragments of memories, both recoverable and forgotten. Initially, we asked her to step on the pieces of paper that symbolized the recoverable memories. Stepping on them, she accurately described their content. Then we asked her to step on a sheet that symbolized one of the blocked memory fragments. Initially, nothing happened, but after 10–20 seconds, the blocked memory fragment began to unfold. In this case, when working with externally oriented trance, we can see the application of the technique of working with the timeline, a spatial metaphor that significantly facilitates the search for memories in the mind.

Hypermnesia

If we are discussing the phenomenon of hypermnesia, it allows us to retrieve not just any memory fragment but its detailed content. For example, during training on the use of hypermnesia in hypnotic suggestion, we invite students to try visualizing a beloved children's book after recreating a hypnotic regression into childhood. They are instructed to open the book to a specific page and attempt to read the text written there. After the training session, they return home and check if they have successfully recalled the specific text indicated on the given page.

Transderivation Search

The process of memory retrieval is one in which a particular sensation or emotion is taken as a starting point to find the desired memory fragment.

Let's provide an interesting example from our practice. During a group psychotherapy session, one of our students mentioned experiencing a strange feeling of nausea when attempting to relax her tense trapezius muscles. We asked her to sit next to us, applied pressure to her trapezius muscles to reproduce the negative sensation, instructed her to close her eyes, and gently induced a light trance state. We then suggested that the sensation she experiences when pressure is applied to her trapezius muscles would guide her into the depths of her memory and reveal the memory fragment from which this sensation originated. When we brought her out of trance, she shared that she recalled when she was ten years old, her parents took her to a masseur who had a strange look in his eyes when working on her. She remembered that the feeling of nausea occurred when he was massaging her. "Most likely, he had a strong sexual attraction toward me," the young woman said.

Positive Hypnotic Hallucinations

The phenomenon of positive hallucinations occurs when a person sees, hears, or feels something that does not exist in reality. For example, they may see an implanted image of an apple on the table, a hovering ball in front of their eyes, or an imaginary person sitting on a chair. The hallucination can be either suggested or spontaneous, depending on the type of suggestion given by the hypnotic suggestor. If the hallucination is auditory, it could be someone's speech, a simple sound, or even a melody. A kinesthetic hallucination may manifest as a sensation of touch, the feeling of the body floating in weightlessness, and so on. Hallucinations can be tentatively categorized as true or false. True hallucination cannot be distinguished from real objects, while false hallucination markedly differs in quality from actual perceptions.

Positive hypnotic illusions differ from hallucinations in that a person perceives, sees, hears, or feels a real object in a distorted manner. For example, a real apple may appear purple, a male voice is perceived as female, or a dry hand feels wet.

Let's provide an example of creating true hallucinations with one of our students during a seminar. We induced a deep hypnotic trance in a student with a hysteroid personality profile. When she reached a sufficient depth of trance and began demonstrating catalepsy and levitation of both hands, we suggested to her that she was traveling ten years into the future. This created an additional trance phenomenon of age progression, where we could project our ideas of the future as sensory experiences. Then we instructed her that with a snap of our fingers, her eyes would open, and while remaining in a trance state, she would see a sphere in front of her that would show her glimpses of her future. We snapped our fingers, and her eyes opened slightly, squinting. It was clear that she was focusing on something in front of her. We then re-induced the trance with closed eyes for a few more minutes, followed by post-hypnotic suggestions, and eventually brought her out of the trance.

After coming out of the trance, she told us about her experience. When she opened her eyes in the trance, she saw a round sphere with fuzzy edges, about 40–50 centimeters in diameter. She looked inside the sphere and saw herself with children and a husband (at the time of hypnosis, she was not married and had no children) on an island. She felt a surge of energy and happiness.

If we continue discussing age progression, we can describe its various variations. For example, Milton Erickson used age progression with patients who didn't know how to achieve a certain life goal. He created a hypnosis session with the patient and progressed them into a hypothetical future where they could achieve that goal. While the patient remained in their subjective representation of the future, the therapist asked them how they had already achieved their goal. The patient, associated with the situation of accomplishment, described in detail how they had achieved it. Upon coming out of trance, Erickson simply relayed to the patient what he had heard during the trance. In this case, we see how information derived from the projection of personal future representations can be utilized.

Another intriguing example is the technique of working with hypnosis on people who are dying from cancer. This is not a method of treating cancer but rather an emotional preparation for the process of dying. Patients were put into a hypnotic trance and then progressed to the moment of death. The goal was for the patient to find their own representation of where their consciousness would reside after death. Then, when the patient progressed to that state, the hypnotherapist would interview them about their experiences, ask them to say goodbye to their loved ones, and let go of the world. Patients who underwent this form of regressive hypnosis underwent significant changes in their attitudes toward the world, themselves, and the process of death and dying, significantly reducing emotional distress.

The technique we used at the time for treating death anxiety in patients was effective. Let's provide a similar example. A 40-year-old woman had been experiencing intense fear during air travel for many years. She often resorted to heavy drinking during flights to numb her anxiety and unease, but even that didn't always help. In our interaction with her, we attempted the following approach. We induced a trance state and recreated a fantasy of an airplane crash that she had experienced. Then, we asked her to imagine a series of dead bodies of people involved in the crash. The next step in working with the trance motif was to have her envision herself lying among the deceased. When this was visualized, we uttered the phrase, "It's all over now." Tears started streaming down the patient's face as she intensely relived the sensation of being beyond the boundary of life. Subsequently, we brought her out of the trance and asked for feedback on her well-being. She felt as if something had been purged from within. A week later, she flew on a plane to visit her daughter in Prague. When she returned and came to see us, she reported flying without fear for the first time in her life.

Similar techniques involving age progression beyond life are not new and have been part of Hindu and Buddhist practices for centuries. The essence of these practices involved meditating on the image of oneself as a deceased individual. Some monks would deliberately visit cemeteries to engage in prolonged contemplation and meditation on the actual bodies of the dead. Indeed, the associated experience of being beyond the threshold removes fear and unease.

In neuro-linguistic programming, a technique called "Old Bones" was developed, utilizing the phenomenon of age progression for individuals seeking advice regarding their current life situations. This technique can be applied both in a hypnotic format and as a pattern without direct hypnotic induction. In either case, the structure of "Old Bones" is a modified version of Milton Erickson's technique involving age progression. With this technique, the patient is induced to believe that they have aged significantly and can, from the perspective of extensive life experience, offer themselves in the past adequate and constructive advice and recommendations.

Age regression

The hypnotic phenomenon of age regression is similar in its creation to age progression, with the exception that the hypnotic suggestion is directed backward in time instead of forward. This phenomenon was a favorite among hypnotherapists in the late 19th and early 20th centuries. Some hypnotherapists even used it as a standardized template, considering it their primary therapeutic tool. Some believed that it was necessary to return the patient to a traumatic experience and evoke a cathartic reaction (J. Breuer), through which a healing effect could be achieved. Others implanted false memories to alleviate a person's suffering (P. Janet), while some helped patients in a state of age regression to complete unfinished business (R. Bender).

We have previously described the cases of J. Breuer and P. Janet in our book. R. Bender, through the technique of completing memories, assisted Vietnam veterans suffering from PTSD. For example, one of his patients experienced painful reminiscences (visual flashbacks) in which he relived the scene of his friend's suicide multiple times. He suffered from severe depression, and during one of his military helicopter flights, he simply jumped out of the door. R. Bender regressed his patient to the traumatic situation and, in a trance, concluded it differently. He suggested to the patient that he had successfully boarded the helicopter and retrieved his friend's body. Then he transported them back to America. The trance visualization of this scene significantly alleviated the patient's emotional suffering.

As Russian psychologist B. Zeigarnik discovered in her research, we are much more likely to hold memories of unfinished or improperly completed events in our memory. R. Bender's work demonstrates how we can help a patient release their attention from a sense of incompleteness through hypnotic techniques. Although this release may not be complete and may differ from literal real-life closure, in the practice of hypnotherapy, we can observe a genuine therapeutic effect solely through trance visualization.

Negative hypnotic hallucination.

Negative visual hallucinations occur in consciousness when a person does not see, hear, or perceive an actual existing object. Nevertheless, even when the phenomenon of negative hallucination is created, the process of perceiving surrounding objects continues to occur; the individual simply loses awareness of what has been perceived. Let's provide an example to clarify

162

this thought further.

Stephen Gilligan shared a story about experiments with creating negative visual hallucinations. Individuals were induced into a hypnotic trance state, and it was suggested that they would negatively hallucinate any furniture in the room. Then they were asked to open their eyes and walk in a straight line toward the opposite wall. On their path, a table was placed. The patient would approach the table but then walk around it. When later questioned about why they deviated from a straight path toward the opposite wall, the patient would respond that they did not know; they simply felt like it. Similar results were obtained with other participants in the experiment. This indicates that the process of perception continues to occur, but on a conscious level, the person is not aware of what they perceive. However, their unconscious reactions still indicate that sensory information continues to reach the brain, be processed, and generate appropriate responses to external stimuli.

A somewhat similar experiment was conducted by doctors with patients suffering from anterograde amnesia. This form of amnesia occurs when a person loses the ability to remember or retain anything after a traumatic experience. All memory before the traumatic event continues to be preserved, as well as the memory of the last 15-20 minutes of the most recent experience. Therefore, after this short period of time, any event falls out of memory and can no longer be consciously recalled. Doctors attempted the following approach. They approached an anterograde amnesic patient, holding a handheld electric shocker in their hand, shook their hand, and simultaneously shocked them. Then they left and returned after half an hour, when the patient had already forgotten about the previous handshake. When they reached out their hand for a handshake again, the patient refused. When asked why they refused, the patient could not formulate a reason for their behavior.

As in the case of hypnotic negative hallucinations and antero-grade amnesia, we can see that conscious control over certain mental processes is lost, but these processes themselves do not disappear, and the unconscious part of the mind continues to adequately react to the world.

Hypnotic phenomena of time illusions

There are various phenomena of time distortion that can occur during trance induction. Some of them occur spontaneously and accompany the trance process, while others can be created through specific suggestions. One of the most commonly encountered trance phenomena is compressed time. It often arises simply as a result of deep immersion in a hypnotic state. And sometimes, the deeper the trance, the stronger the compression of time. Compression usually occurs at a rate of 2–3 times per second. For example, if a patient was in a trance state for 30 minutes, upon exiting, they may comment that it felt like only 10 minutes had passed. Observing patients experiencing such time compression, we have found that almost all of these trance sessions were emotionally rich, possessed significant therapeutic potential, and led to constructive changes. The presence of the time compression phenomenon, in our opinion, indicates a deep rapport between the hypnotherapist and the patient. It reflects the patient's internal readiness for positive transformation. Often, during the manifestation of time compression, hypnotic amnesia can spontaneously occur for the duration of the trance induction.

The phenomenon of extended time is encountered much

less frequently and, in our opinion, is a consequence of the patient's inability to integrate an internal conflict that may be unexpressed in the conscious realm during trance induction. Typically, this phenomenon is accompanied by negative emotions, ominous premonitions, and dark or black-and-white images. After a trance session with such time distortion, patients often feel uncomfortable. However, despite this discomfort, this phenomenon provides indications of a significant internal conflict that requires additional psychotherapeutic exploration.

There is an interesting story about Milton Erickson's work with a patient who had a very peculiar symptom. She would go to sleep and dream that she was going on a vacation by the sea and spending many days there. The dream was wonderful, except for one drawback: she wouldn't wake up in reality and continued sleeping for several days at a time while her consciousness was enjoying the vacation. Once, she was out of contact with her loved ones for over a week. When they went to her home, they found her peacefully asleep. She had been sleeping continuously for over a week, and her body was in terrible condition. She was taken to the hospital and later referred to Milton Erickson for consultation, seeking his assistance. The legend goes that Erickson worked with her only once, using a hypnotic trance, in which he suggested that she would be able to continue having similar dream journeys in the future, where she could spend a week or more, but in reality, it would only take a couple of hours.

In essence, one could say that he taught her to expand time in her dreams during trance. We have never encountered a similar phenomenon of hyperextended time in the process of hypnotic induction. However, we have observed this phenomenon in the dreams of some patients. They would describe dreams in which they lived for several weeks, months, or even years, and upon waking up, it felt as if they remembered many days spent in some other place. It is worth noting that descriptions of such dream phenomena are very rare. Additionally, it is interesting to note that after dreams with hyperextended time, people experience intense and unusual sensations and emotions, which are more often positive than negative.

In our observations, the phenomenon of absent time did not spontaneously manifest during the trance process, although we acknowledge that it could potentially occur. To understand what this phenomenon represents, it is important to note that for each person, the representation of time is always at the level of bodily sensations. In other words, we deal with the perception of time. We feel that time is passing. Each of us may have our own subjective representation of it. And, naturally, any sensation in the body can be turned on or off using hypnotic inductions. The phenomenon of absent time, in its form, resembles hypnotic analgesia, where we disable sensitivity to pain in a specific area or throughout the entire body.

Hypnotic phenomena of alternative personalities

Our personality consists of fragments, different parts that have been formed during different periods of personality development. These parts interact with each other in a specific way, like employees of the same company. Some parts are more friendly towards each other, while others are not. Each of these parts can have different values and beliefs.

For example, one part may prioritize work and career advancement, another may prioritize friends and socializing, and yet another may prioritize spirituality and self-development. Our integrated personality is a compromise among these parts. In mentally healthy individuals, there is always a core personality that governs the other subpersonalities. Volitional control emanates from this core personality. Some subpersonalities may be stable, while others may be traumatized. A stable subpersonality is always in effective interaction with the core personality.

For example, if the core personality primarily manages work and career and one of the subpersonalities is focused on friendships and leisure activities, and both of these parts are stable, then the person can effectively integrate these aspects into their life without experiencing internal conflict. However, if one of the parts is traumatized, its manifestation can lead to internal conflict because what one part desires may be completely contradictory to the desires of another part. For instance, the work-oriented part may insist that "you're not earning enough; you need to work more; you can't afford to rest." In response, the part associated with leisure activities may say, "forget about work, let's meet up with friends and have a good time." If one part is significantly stronger than the other, the weaker part is repressed in the unconscious. However, when two parts are roughly equal in strength and the person cannot choose one over the other, they experience internal conflict, which can only be resolved by finding a compromise between these two parts. This is an example of a possible neurotic disorder.

It is important to understand that conflicts can arise among multiple parts of the personality. Sometimes, it is not just a conflict but a full-fledged struggle. In such cases, neurotic disorders can develop into borderline personality disorders or psychoses. In mild personality disorders, the conflict can be consciously recognized. In more severe cases, one part of the personality may have no awareness of the other parts.

In some instances, multiple core personalities can coexist within an individual's consciousness. In certain psychiatric cases, clinicians have identified up to 70 core personalities, which can vary in age, race, and gender. However, these are critical forms of multiple personality disorder. In milder forms, there may be only 2–3 personalities of the same gender, age, and race, sometimes without a change in name.

As an example, let's consider a case from an American clinic involving a woman with symptoms of multiple personality disorder. She had two core personalities with different names. During the psychiatric evaluation, the doctors conducted a blood test and discovered that she had diabetes. After some time, when she transitioned into her alternative personality, another blood test was conducted, and an astonishing finding emerged—the second personality did not have diabetes at all. The test was repeated several times while the patient was in different personalities, consistently confirming that the symptoms of diabetes manifested exclusively in one personality.

We are not aware of similar observations or examples, and it would be incorrect to make generalizations based on a single case. However, we can hypothesize that any physical or mental illness is a reflection of a personality disorder. As part of the mosaic of assertions, we can provide an example of a belief existing in psychospiritual and psychotherapeutic circles that any illness is a reflection of a moral violation. Through analyzing numerous cases in our work with patients, we find multiple confirmations of this belief.

Hypnotic suggestion often provides unique opportunities

for working with such a disorder. In hypnosis, one can communicate with any personality, understand them, activate or deactivate them, and even attempt to reconcile different parts with each other.

When it comes to individuals who do not suffer from multiple personality disorder, it is possible to temporarily create the phenomenon of multiple personalities under hypnosis. This can be done for experimental purposes or with psychotherapeutic intentions.

For example, the technique of interacting with different parts of the personality in hypnosis involves directly addressing one of them, saying, "Now I would like to speak with your joyful personality," or sad, or anxious, whichever you prefer. After the statement, the person usually transitions into an alternative personality, and communication can be established with that part.

For instance, starting with the phrase "I welcome you," the part responds in some way, and the dialogue continues. Sometimes, upon emerging from trance, the person may continue to remember their conversation with the alternative personality, while other times, the dialogue is amnesic.

During the transition to the alternative personality, the suggestible individual's nonverbal communication almost always changes. Their posture, gestures, bearing, tone, tempo, depth, volume of voice, and so on may differ from the main personality. What an artificially induced alternative personality can express may be unfamiliar to the primary personality. Hence, this technique can be used for hypnoanalysis.

We provided a simple example of implementing this technique in the section of the book dedicated to the schizophrenic accentuation of personality, where we described our interaction with a patient suffering from paranoid schizophrenic personality disorder.

For instance, hysteric personalities, when using this technique, can provide vivid representations of their parts. Representatives of other psychopathological profiles usually display less intense manifestations of different parts of their personality. However, everything is connected to the intensities of emotions hidden within them.

It is also worth noting that different parts of the personality may have different psychopathological profiles. One part may be psychopathic, while another may be epileptoid. This information should be taken into account during the psychopathological profiling of the personality.

Stage hypnotists can create interesting variations of this phenomenon.

The phenomenon of induced animal role

For example, inducing a person to transition into an animal role, such as a cat, dog, or any other animal. After appropriate suggestion, the person begins to exhibit behavior characteristic of the suggested animal image while in an externally oriented trance state for a certain period of time. Sometimes, consciousness forms amnesia during this period.

Hypnotic phenomena of awakening creative abilities

Numerous experiments have been conducted using hypnosis to activate latent creative abilities in individuals. A Ukrainian psychiatrist has demonstrated examples of implementing this technique on volunteers whom he hypnotized, suggesting that they become famous artist or musician, and then allowing them to draw or play musical instruments. People who underwent such techniques were often amazed when they viewed or listened to the results of their activity. According to their accounts, the induced and expressed skills in hypnosis were previously inaccessible to them. These experiments were conducted not only by medical professionals but also by stage hypnotists for the purpose of entertaining the audience. The essence remained unchanged.

The recreation of creative ability can be divided into two main practices. The first involves inducing an alternative personality, often a known one, who possessed or possesses certain creative abilities. The second involves inducing the creation or enhancement of creative skill without altering the personality. In our opinion, the first practice is much more effective. However, this hypothesis still needs to be tested.

When examining the activities of artists, musicians, writers, and representatives of other forms of creativity, one can discover their specific methods of self-inducing trance states to enhance their creative abilities. An interesting method was employed by the artist Salvador Dali. He would sit in front of a blank canvas, take a spoon in his hand, hold it over a plate, and wait until he started to fall asleep. When this happened, he would drop the spoon, awakening due to the sound of its fall. Afterward, he would take a brush and attempt to depict on the canvas the unusual images that appeared in his consciousness on the border between wakefulness and sleep. The "Salvador Dali creativity pattern" can be easily reproduced without a spoon and plate, but with the help of hypnotic induction. However, the images obtained through this method will likely differ from those in dreams. The states of trance and sleep are significantly different, even at the level of brain rhythms—measurable electrical oscillations. Let's briefly delve into this topic and indicate the frequencies at which the brain operates when a person is asleep, in a hypnotic trance, or awake. We will discuss the following brain rhythms: delta rhythm, theta rhythm, alpha rhythm, beta rhythm, and gamma rhythm.

- **Delta rhythm**. The frequency of oscillations ranges from 1 to 4 Hz with an amplitude of 20–200 μV. This rhythm is associated with restorative processes that naturally occur during sleep. An excess of delta rhythm during wakefulness predisposes to the impairment of various cognitive functions.

- **Theta rhythm**. The frequency of oscillations in this rhythm ranges from 4 to 8 Hz with an amplitude of 20-100 μV. It is registered in the frontal area and hippocampus. Activation of the theta rhythm occurs during the transition from relaxed wakefulness to light drowsiness. This rhythm is specifically observed in individuals in a state of hypnotic trance and other forms of altered states of consciousness. Theta rhythm often transitions into delta rhythm naturally. It can also naturally arise during chronic fatigue and stress. This rhythm is sometimes referred to as the "twilight" rhythm, which serves as the most appropriate metaphor for its function.

- **Alpha rhythm**. The frequency of oscillations varies within 8–13 Hz with an amplitude of 5-100 μV. It is predominantly registered in the occipital and temporal regions of the brain. This rhythm is associated with a relaxed state of wakefulness that occurs when we close our eyes and begin to relax. A decrease in alpha waves occurs when a person actively engages in tasks requiring visualization. Additionally, a decrease can be caused by emotions such as anger, anxiety, fear, or worry.

· **Beta rhythm**. The frequency of oscillations ranges from 14 to 40 Hz, with oscillation amplitudes reaching up to 20 μV but typically ranging from 3 to 7 μV in a normal state. It is registered in the frontal and central gyri, as well as extending to the posterior central and frontal gyri. This brain rhythm is associated with a state of active wakefulness, cognitive processes, and focused problem-solving. It diminishes during motor activity and tactile stimulation and is more active with open eyes. An increase in beta rhythm is a response to stressful factors.

· **Gamma rhythm**. The frequency of oscillations varies within 30−100 Hz, with typical oscillation amplitudes up to 15 μV. It is registered in the precentral, frontal, parietal, and temporal regions of the cerebral cortex. The gamma rhythm is observed during tasks that require maximum concentration and focus.

From delta rhythm to gamma rhythm, we observe a gradual increase in the frequency of the rhythm from 1 to 100 Hz, accompanied by subsequent changes in the functional characteristics of the brain.

Inducing theta rhythm in human brain activity opens the doors to its unconscious structures while maintaining the ability to interact with them. This can lead to healing trance states, the activation of extraordinary creative abilities, and the control of physiological body functions and states of consciousness. The specific method of generating this theta rhythm becomes a matter of personal choice. The entire spectrum of techniques, from shamanic chanting and dancing to Ericksonian hypnosis and generative trance, can be suitable.

Brain rhythms	Frequency of oscillations	States
Delta rhythm	1-4 Hz	Sleep, narcotic sleep, deep sedation
Theta rhythm	4-8 Hz	Altered states of consciousness, trance, hypnosis, exhaustion
Alpha rhythm	8-13 Hz	Relaxed wakefulness
Beta rhythm	14-40 Hz	Active wakefulness
Gamma rhythm	30-100 Hz	Hyperactive wakefulness

Brain Rhythms

The human brain exhibits various rhythmic patterns known as brain rhythms. These rhythms are characterized by their specific frequency of oscillations and are associated with distinct states of consciousness. Understanding these brain rhythms is crucial to comprehending the complex workings of the mind.

The delta rhythm, with a frequency ranging from 1 to 4 Hz, is primarily observed during sleep, narcotic sleep, and deep sedation. It represents a state of profound mental rest and restoration.

The theta rhythm, oscillating between 4 and 8 Hz, is linked to altered states of consciousness such as trance, hypnosis, and even exhaustion. During these states, the mind enters a realm where perception and awareness undergo significant shifts.

Moving on to the alpha rhythm, which ranges from 8 to 13 Hz, we enter the domain of relaxed wakefulness. This rhythm becomes prominent when we close our eyes, seeking relaxation and tranquility. It reflects a state of calm and serenity, often associated with a meditative or reflective mindset.

Transitioning to higher frequencies, we encounter the beta rhythm, with oscillations spanning from 14 to 40 Hz. This rhythm dominates during active wakefulness, when the mind is alert, focused, and engaged in cognitive tasks. Beta rhythm signifies heightened mental activity and concentration.

Lastly, we arrive at the gamma rhythm, which encompasses frequencies between 30 and 100 Hz. This rhythm corresponds to a state of hyperactive wakefulness, characterized by intense mental engagement, heightened sensory processing, and maximal concentration. It is prevalent during tasks that demand exceptional cognitive capabilities.

By deciphering and comprehending the intricacies of these brain rhythms, we can gain profound insights into the functioning of the human mind. Exploring their interplay and significance contributes to our understanding of consciousness, cognition, and the vast potential of our mental capacities.

Hypnotic Phenomenon of Motor Analog Signaling

During the process of hypnotic work, the human body can exhibit various motor signals. These can manifest as slight tremors or twitches in the hands, legs, and head, as well as spontaneous changes in their position. Each of these unconscious movements holds significance and reflects changes in trance states. In order to transform these subtle motor movements into a fully-fledged language of communication, the establishment of specific hypnotic frames becomes necessary. These frames enable the unconscious suggestee to express themselves in an orderly and clear manner.

It is likely that Leslie LeCron was one of the first to apply motor analog signaling in the 1950s and 1960s in America. In his work with patients, he created a simple framework for the unconscious patient to respond to the psychotherapist. The framework was as follows: "If your unconscious wants to answer 'yes,' let it raise the index finger of the right hand. If it wants to answer 'no,' let it raise the left finger." Once this framework was established, the psychotherapist would begin asking questions to the unconscious patient, carefully observing the resulting movements. The movement of a specific finger would indicate a particular response from the unconscious. Often, the patient may not be aware of their own finger movements, as they occur unconsciously.

LeCron initially proposed using such a form of communication with the unconscious for hypnoanalysis, which involves uncovering the root cause of existing symptoms. He also suggested a set of basic questions that could be asked of the patient during hypnoanalysis, utilizing motor analog signaling.

These questions are now known as "**LeCron's Keys**"

1. **Conflict**. Is the symptom a result of any past conflict? This question can be posed in two forms, using the terms "external conflict" and "internal conflict." External conflict refers to any altercation, fight, or similar events. Internal conflict encompasses dilemmas in decision-making, the inability to make a choice, conflicts of conscience, and actions.

2. **Motivation**. Is there any hidden internal motivation that leads to the emergence of the symptom? The term "positive intention" is commonly used in psychotherapy today. Behind any symptom, there may be a concealed benefit. Although the person may not consciously understand the cause of the problem, analyzing their life situation can reveal that they are not receiving something important without the symptom. A simple example would be an elderly person who frequently falls ill and receives a lot of attention from their relatives. If the illness were absent, they might lose the necessary attention.

3. **Suggestion effect**. Is the symptom a result of any past suggestion? Indeed, several symptoms arise as a consequence of negative suggestions made to us during childhood or other periods of time. Many inappropriate beliefs about one's sexual life are passed down by mothers and grandmothers to their daughters and granddaughters. Let's recall a case where a patient described how her grandmother would "brainwash" her during childhood. The grandmother would take her to the window, point to an arch in the building, and tell her, "Do you see, my dear, one evening when you're walking there, five boys

will catch you, pin you down, and one of them will violate you." Such suggestions do not necessarily determine a person's life, but they certainly have an impact, reflecting changes in certain aspects of behavior.

4. **Elements of "organic speech**." Is the symptom a result of using "organic speech"? This point requires further clarification. In our speech, we often employ verbal metaphors that can directly influence bodily sensations, bypassing their figurative or abstract meaning. Examples of such metaphors include phrases like "Why are you so sour?", "You'll break your neck," "Lose your head," "Your hands are growing from the wrong place," "Everything is twisted," and so on. Theoretically, each metaphor used in the right context and at the right time can have an impact on physical and mental well-being. This was believed by Lekron, who once shared a case involving a lawyer who complained of a bad taste in his mouth. Despite undergoing medical examinations that revealed no underlying illnesses, the symptom persisted. Lekron employed motor analog signaling with the client to uncover the cause of the symptom, and a positive response was linked to the element of "organic speech." Subsequently, Lekron began questioning the patient about whether he or someone in his surroundings had used words related to a bad taste shortly before the onset of the symptom. Indeed, the patient quickly found an answer to this question. He revealed that during that time, he was handling a case in court, defending a person whom he knew to be guilty. However, he managed to prove the person's complete innocence in court, which

caused him to experience feelings of guilt. He would then mention to acquaintances that the case had "bad taste." Such self-suggestion, intertwined with feelings of guilt or shame, could manifest as a symptom. In this case, the use of such words provides the unconscious mind with an alternative means of communicating with the conscious sphere about what it represses or suppresses. On the other hand, it should be noted that, in our opinion, if there is no repression or suppression of negative emotions in a specific life situation, the likelihood of these types of phrases manifesting as symptoms is quite low.

5. **Identification**. Is the onset of the symptom a result of identification with another person? Sometimes, a symptom arises from our identification with a close individual. On an unconscious level, our conscience can "compel" us to share their fate in order to satisfy our social instinct. The topic of symptom inheritance through identification is extensively explored and interpreted by systemic family and transgenerational therapy. We will not delve into this topic in detail here, as it deserves a separate book.

6. **Masochism**. Is the symptom a result of masochistic tendencies? It would be more accurate to refer to this point as the "need for self-punishment." "Guilt is a sense of balance," said Bert Hellinger, a German psychotherapist, during one of his seminars. When we commit an act that goes against our conscience, we seek ways to balance the "amoral" action with a symptom that may restrain us from engaging in similar actions in the

future. Thus, a symptom is always a form of unconscious resistance to our own actions or the actions of individuals with whom we have a psycho-emotional connection.

7. **Painful experiences from the past**. Is the symptom a consequence of painful experiences from the past? This point highlights the connection between experiencing negative sensations and emotions from the past and the current symptom. Let's provide a simple example: During a consultation with a psychoanalyst, a patient confessed that she had a strong internal, unconscious prohibition against using swear words. After some time, they discovered the cause of her symptom in the patient's childhood. When she was around 5 years old, she over-heard profanity on the street and then decided to share her discovery with her mother during dinner. In response, her mother took her to the bathroom and washed her mouth with household soap. This form of upbringing may not be ecologically sound, but it seems to have been quite effective.

Naturally, there can be many more keys to uncovering the cause of a symptom than those listed by Lekron. However, they would involve questions that provide further details on a specific point from his list.

If we return to the general topic of motor analog signaling, it is worth mentioning that it is not necessary to limit the variety of unconscious responses to only "yes" or "no." Different finger movements can be assigned to responses such as "don't know," "don't want to talk about it," "you don't need to know that right now," and so on. Similarly, you can work with a list of different answers. For example, you can ask the unconscious mind, "What would be the best activity for me right now?" with options like a) "Work," b) "Take a walk," c) "Eat," d) "Sleep." In this case, each answer option can be assigned to different fingers of one hand, or other answer options can be used.

An interesting application of motor analog signaling is found in Neuro-Linguistic Programming (NLP) and the technique of six-step reframing, where the therapist uses unconscious responses not only to gather specific information from the past but also to initiate or stop certain mental and neuro-physiological processes in the present. For example, asking the unconscious mind, "Creative part of the personality, can you find new ways to manifest the positive intention of the part of the personality responsible for the symptom?" vividly illustrates this example. As a result, the number of questions that can be asked expands significantly. Let's refer to these types of *questions as process keys*. Here are some examples of these keys:

· Unconscious mind, can you immerse consciousness in a deep hypnotic trance?
· Unconscious mind, can you show the cause of the symp-tom?
· Unconscious mind, can you initiate the process of psy-chotherapeutic transformation?
· Creative part of the personality, can you demonstrate a variety of constructive solutions to the situation?
· Part of the personality responsible for the symptom, can you show what you truly want to achieve?
· Wise part of the personality, can you reveal any new mean-ing for the existing situation to help me better understand

it?

And so on. The questions can be very diverse, and their combination can create individual psychotherapeutic algorithms.

By the way, it is worth mentioning that motor analog signaling does not necessarily have to be performed after inducing a hypnotic trance. The process of verbal communication with the unconscious mind and its parts itself creates a trance-like process. Therefore, essentially, it is only necessary to establish the framework of therapeutic communication, assign response options to the fingers, and begin the communication itself. However, for some individuals, performing this phenomenon after a trance induction may be more effective.

Hypnotic phenomenon of jactation

This is a relatively rare trance phenomenon that sometimes occurs during public performances by stage hypnotists who use prolonged monotonic types of hypnotic induction. In this case, a person's body may start rhythmically swaying from side to side or making circular movements clockwise and counterclockwise. Sometimes there can be an uncontrolled rhythmic raising and lowering of the arms. Similar phenomena have been observed during group hypnosis sessions with Ukrainian hypnotist V. Kashpirovsky. Based on our observations, the usual type of trance induction does not spontaneously produce this phenomenon. However, when we attempted to recreate Kashpirovsky's working style in a hypnosis laboratory, we found that some participants started exhibiting similar hypnotic rocking phenomena.

Hypnotic taste and smell illusions

This hypnotic phenomenon creates taste distortions when consuming food in a trance state. It is difficult to trace the original context in which this phenomenon was first practiced, whether in a clinical or stage setting. However, it is more commonly practiced by stage hypnotists for entertainment purposes. Most often, during a hypnotic trance, the suggestion is given that the person will now taste a delicious sweet fruit or something similar, and then they are given a bitter onion or a sour lemon to try. If the suggestion is successful, the true taste is not perceived at all. The person can eat a bitter onion, crying from the onion's smell irritating their eyes, but at the same time, they can comment on its amazing taste qualities without showing any facial muscle reaction to the bitterness. Naturally, along with this, a hypnotic illusion of smell is also created. This phenomenon can also be turned into taste and olfactory hallucinations by suggesting to the person that they are holding a fruit that does not actually exist.

Hypnotic paralysis

The phenomenon of hypnotic paralysis, in the overwhelming majority of cases, requires intentional induction. Although we have seen a few cases where it occurred spontaneously in hysterical patients during the creation of catalepsy of the arm. In such cases, while remaining in a hypnotic trance, the person retains the ability to communicate and can even stand up and move around, but their arm remains frozen and paralyzed. Willpower does not lead to the removal of paralysis. In other cases, paralysis of the hands and the entire body is created through specific hypnotic inductions.

Hypnotic phenomenon of rebirth

183

In describing the phenomenon of hypnotic regression, we have already touched upon this topic when discussing the work of Bert Hellinger. In a hypnotic state, the experience of rebirth can be induced by regressing the patient to the moment of their birth. To stimulate association with this memory, it is necessary to perform bodily imitative actions. For example, placing the patient in a hypnotic state on a mat in the fetal position. Then, with the assistance of a helper standing beside the patient, they embrace the patient, simulating contact with the mother in the intrauterine state. Subsequently, spasms of the uterus are imitated by the helper applying pressure to the patient's body from all sides. Following this, pulling movements are made to evoke neurophysiological associations with the process of traversing the birth canal.

Formally, this description corresponds to the technique of V. Reich-O. Rank, "Birth of a New Child," which was demonstrated to us by Alexander Danilov. The psychotherapeutic aspect of this practice is based on the theories of Otto Rank, who introduced the concept of "birth trauma" into psychoanalysis and hypnoanalysis. According to O. Rank, during the process of birth, a person undergoes a significant amount of emotionally and physically painful states, which are then suppressed and can potentially contribute to neurotic and even psychotic processes in the individual's personality. Re-experiencing this event can lead to catharsis—a psychoemotional cleansing of consciousness from these emotions and feelings.

In a section of the book dedicated to the manic-depressive profile of personality, we commented on our observations regarding the fact that difficult and problematic childbirth can potentially lead to the formation of a manic-depressive accent in the personality or even its full-fledged psychotic manifestation in the future. Therefore, in our opinion, in such cases, the hypnotic re-experiencing of birth can possess exceptional psychotherapeutic potential.

Let us present our observations in a slightly different trance context. During holotropic breathing sessions, patients some-times regress on their own to the moment of birth and begin intensely re-experiencing it without any external involvement.

Once, we observed a patient during holotropic breathing who became associated with the birthing process, and she believed that she was the one giving birth and that the baby was emerging through her birth canal. However, she had never experienced childbirth before. We interpreted this case as an associated re-experiencing of her own birth through the mother's image. We have not encountered any other similar cases, so we refrain from making any generalizing statements on this matter.

Hypnotic Phenomenon of Regression into Past Lives

Russian psychiatrist and hypnotherapist V. Raikov practiced a fascinating form of hypnotherapy with alcoholics in the 1960s and 1970s. By inducing them into a state of hypnotic trance, he regressed them along the timeline, first into early childhood, and then suggested that they transition from their current life to their past incarnation in their consciousness. Patients began to recall and share their experiences in this state, describing who they were and what they did. V. Raikov then suggested that they look from there into their future incarnation, where they would die, be reborn, and descend into alcoholism in the next life. The realization of this was often shocking for the patients. According to V. Raikov, many of those who experienced this process eventually quit drinking or significantly reduced their alcohol consumption.

Many years ago, together with my students, we experimented with inducing the experience of past incarnations through hypnotic suggestion and discovered a remarkable phenomenon. The majority of students who reenacted this phenomenon easily regressed into the experience of their past incarnation and provided detailed feedback about who they were and what they did.

It is difficult to determine the nature of this phenomenon. Rationalistic reductionists would argue that we are dealing with fantasies of the patient's unconscious mind. Transpersonal psychologists, on the other hand, would claim that we are dealing with genuine experiences of past incarnations. At present, we cannot fully confirm or refute either viewpoint. Therefore, let us focus on the fact that such experiences can be reproduced, analyzed, and integrated into other forms of therapeutic work, yielding significant therapeutic results. Let me provide an example from the psychotherapeutic work of Stanislav Grof, who utilized the method of holotropic breathwork. One of his patients had been plagued by a psychosomatic symptom for the past 20 years. She suffered from persistent frontal sinusitis and maxillary sinusitis, which did not improve regardless of the treatments she received. During a holotropic breathwork session, she regressed into a memory of one of her past incarnations and recalled being a young woman in an English medieval village, regarded as a witch by the villagers. They caught her, tied her to a board, and submerged her head into the water of a lake, resulting in her death. In the holotropic trance, she fully relived the process of her death. After some time following the psychotherapeutic session, she began to notice that the symptoms of frontal sinusitis and maxillary sinusitis started to recede. The symptoms disappeared and never returned. Stanislav Grof's books contain several similar cases of working with patients and their regressions into past lives.

Based on our observations and the observations of other psychotherapists who have employed this phenomenon in therapeutic practice, we can affirm its ability to produce a powerful therapeutic effect, sometimes unattainable through other hypnotic methods.

It is worth mentioning our findings in working with this phenomenon. Following the concept of regression, we attempted to recreate the phenomenon of hypnotic reincarnational progression in a hypnotic laboratory with students.

Hypnotic reincarnational progression

We simply induced students into a hypnotic state and then suggested to them that they were becoming associated with their future incarnation. Similar to the previous phenomenon of hypnotic reincarnational regression, most of our students began to re-experience experiences not related to their own personality. Some did so superficially, while others provided highly detailed accounts. Interestingly, we observed a physiological phenomenon in individuals who were in this state and provided feedback on what was happening to them. The more detailed information they commented on, the faster their pulse and breathing became, and they experienced trembling in their hands and sometimes throughout their entire body. We cannot fully interpret such vegetative reactions. However, it can be assumed that during the reproduction of this phenomenon, several areas of the brain are activated. To fully confirm this assumption, it would be necessary to repeat this experiment using MRI equipment.

By activating this hypnotic phenomenon, we initiate unconscious processes of intensive analysis of existing experiences and the projection of assumptions about what they might lead to in future incarnations, assuming that such incarnations exist. However, it is important to note that these projections may be influenced by our desires and fears. In any case, we have found that the material obtained after such hypnoanalysis possesses significant psychotherapeutic value and can be used in the process of psychotherapy.

Phenomenon of false hypnotic paralysis

During hypnosis, you may encounter not only the phenomenon of complete hypnotic paralysis but also its false variant. What does it entail? The patient is aware that they are in a trance and theoretically capable of moving, but a volitional impulse is formed in their consciousness, making them unwilling to move. When prompted by the hypnotist to try to overcome the paralysis on their own, the patient usually manages to do so after several attempts, typically taking 5–20 seconds. This indicates that a certain form of paralysis did exist but was in a more controllable state. When patients who successfully emerged from this state voluntarily provided feedback, they described the process of emerging as similar to attempting to break free from sticky shackles or making progress in a viscous swamp.

Vectors of hypnotic phenomena

Positive hallucinations (illusions)	Negative hallucinations (illusions)
Catalepsy (paralysis)	Levitation (motor analog signaling)
Hyperesthesia	Anesthesia
Hypermnesia	Amnesia
Age progression	Age regression

16

The Use of Hypnotic Phenomena in Psychotherapeutic Practice

In psychotherapeutic practice, there have always been a range of phenomena that have been and will continue to be beloved tools of therapists. These include hypnotic progression and regression, catalepsy, levitation of the hands, and motor analog signaling.

Indeed, these phenomena can be more than sufficient for the treatment of various conditions. However, this does not mean that other phenomena cannot be used as psychotherapeutic tools.

Hypnotic phenomena serve various purposes within the hypnotic trance.

Hypnotic phenomena can serve as clear indicators that the trance has been induced and the patient is receptive to suggestions.

Different phenomena can act as diagnostic criteria for assessing the depth of the induced hypnotic trance and the patient's ability to reach such depths. This, in turn, can provide valuable insights into the patient's specific psychopathological profile. Only individuals belonging to certain psychopathological profiles are capable of fully reproducing certain hypnotic phenomena. For instance, we have observed genuine negative hallucinations exclusively in individuals with a hysteroid profile.

Hypnotic phenomena can trigger changes in the patient's consciousness. For example, during a trance state, the client's arm may be lifted, inducing catalepsy. The hypnotherapist then establishes a framework for change, suggesting that the arm will gradually descend, controlled by impulses from the unconscious. As the arm lowers, a pleasant, warm sensation of joy and happiness increasingly arises in the patient's consciousness. Additionally, one can introduce the criterion of touching the leg with the hand, explaining that when the hand reaches the leg, a new and unusual healing process will initiate in the patient's consciousness. The specific unfolding of events during the lowering of the arm and the touch of the knee can be tailored according to your preference. Furthermore, an alternative approach can involve not lowering the arm from catalepsy but initiating the phenomenon of hand levitation. In this case, we can suggest allowing the unconscious mind to spontaneously move the hand in space, and while the hand levitates, the wise part of your personality will explore new ways to solve the existing challenge.

Ernest Rossi, one of Milton Erickson's closest students, demonstrated another interesting variation in the use of catalepsy and levitation of the hand in a psychotherapeutic context. This technique was later named "Ernest Rossi's Hands."

The execution of the technique is as follows: First, the hypnotherapist identifies the symptom they will work with.

Then, a trance is induced, during which catalepsy is created in the patient's hands. Next, the hypnotherapist verbally associates the patient's right hand with the existing symptom and the left hand with the potential solution existing in the unconscious. A hypnotic induction is then given to prompt the patient's unconscious to begin moving the hands slowly and spontaneously in a trance state. As the hands move, existing unconscious resources that can be used to address and treat the symptom are awakened. The hands start moving; they may travel through space and interact with each other. Often, at the end of the movement, they come together, symbolizing the point of finding an acceptable solution at the conscious or unconscious level. However, there are cases where the hands do not come together and even move apart, indicating the patient's internal resistance to finding a solution. In such cases, it is necessary to either continue the hypnotic session by adding specific interventions that can help activate the correct path to finding a solution or to bring the patient out of the trance, discuss possible causes of unconscious resistance, and attempt to understand them at the conscious level. Then, the technique can be attempted again.

"**Ernest Rossi's Hands**" can be a universal technique applicable to almost any type of symptom during hypnotic work. Based on our observations, this practice has shown good results in working with addictive behaviors. The only important aspect of this form of hypnotic work is the activation of full catalepsy in the hands and their subsequent unconscious movement. In some cases, the movement may be intuitive and semi-conscious, but its effectiveness is diminished. This practice represents an expanded form of working with motor analog signaling, where the unconscious creates an external representation of internal change processes through the movement of the patient's hands.

One very interesting way of using the hypnotic phenomenon in trance is as a metaphor for change and transformation. An example of such work was shared with us during one of the seminars by Alexander Danilov, who discovered a fascinating form of utilizing hypnotic hand catalepsy in the treatment of male erectile dysfunction.

Danilov would induce the patient into a hypnotic trance and then create catalepsy in the hand, keeping it in a vertical position with a clenched fist. He would then suggest to the patient a comparison between the cataleptic hand and the ability of the penis to achieve a similar state. Thus, the hand in catalepsy became a neurophysiological metaphor for the erectile function of male genitalia.

This example demonstrates how different phenomena can be used as metaphors in trance work. Let's provide analogies with other phenomena.

For instance, the hypnotic phenomenon of anesthesia can be employed to address emotionally traumatic situations. To do so, the patient is regressed to the problematic emotional context, followed by the induction of the anesthesia phe-nomenon and its testing by applying pressure to a pain point or pricking the skin with a needle. Afterward, an analogy is drawn between the emotional sphere and pain sensitivity, making the anesthesia metaphor a representation of insensitivity to psychotraumatic experiences.

The cataleptic bridge phenomenon can serve as a powerful metaphor for resilience in the face of life's difficulties. The working strategy can be similar to the previous example. The patient is either progressed into or regressed into the desired context, the cataleptic bridge phenomenon is created, and it is associated with the necessary process or phenomenon.

Visual hallucinations can be an excellent metaphor for the ability to see a way out of a situation when others cannot. Taste illusions can serve as a metaphor for changing the perception of a situation.

By analogy with the examples mentioned above, any hypnotic phenomenon can be transformed into a metaphor for transformation. For ease of use, let's describe an algorithm using hypnotic phenomena as metaphors for transformation.

The structure of utilizing hypnotic phenomena in therapy practice is as follows:

1. Identify the problematic context.
2. Select a hypnotic phenomenon whose metaphor can provide a solution in this context.
3. Induce trance.
4. Associate with the problematic context.
5. Recreate the chosen hypnotic phenomenon.
6. Associate the hypnotic phenomenon with the problematic context, making it a metaphor for transformation.
7. Provide post-hypnotic suggestions.
8. Bring the patient out of a trance.

Certainly, it is worth mentioning that not all phenomena can be reproduced with every patient. It is best to start training in the application of this practice with simpler phenomena and explore in which cases their metaphors for symptom work can be most applicable.

The more difficult it is to reproduce a phenomenon in trance work, the stronger its metaphor for transformation is. Although this is only a hypothesis that is challenging to confirm or refute.

Even if you can only elicit one elementary phenomenon in a patient, such as catalepsy of the hand, using cause-and-effect language, you can integrate it into a certain part of the transformative trance process.

In this book, we have explored the History and Theory of Hypnosis.

In the next book **Hypnotherapy Training: A Guide for Practicing Hypnotherapists** we will delve into the practical aspects of hypnosis. We will examine the levels of hypnotic trance, various styles of hypnotic work, the structural elements of the process, gain an understanding of how the human neuromediator system functions during hypnosis, and engage in a dozen practical exercises to effectively master the skills of a hypnotherapist.

BONUS: Your Free Gifts

Use QR code or link <u>psychemaster.com/psychology-and-psychotherapy-books-series</u> to **receive a free eBook "Psychotherapy Introduction"** from the author, plus links to online **psychological tests** and quizzes.

These resources will guide you in evaluating your well-being and deciding whether to consult a **mental health professional**. You can complete each test in under five minutes and receive immediate results.

Bibliography

1. Nevsky, M.P. The Influence of Unconditioned Stimuli on Brain Electrical Activity in Hypnosis with the Suggestion of Insensitivity to Them. Neuropathology and Psychiatry (Collection of scientific works of the regional psychoneurological hospital and Chelyabinsk branch of the All-Union Scientific Society of Neuropathologists and Psychiatrists). Chelyabinsk, 1960. pp. 271–281.
2. Nevsky, M.P. The Influence of Conditioned (Verbal) Stimuli on Brain Electrical Activity in Hypnosis. Neuropathology and Psychiatry (Collection of scientific works of the regional psychoneurological hospital and Chelyabinsk branch of the All-Union Scientific Society of Neuropathologists and Psychiatrists). Chelyabinsk, 1960. pp. 263–269.
3. Platonov, K.I. Issues of Psychotherapy in Obstetrics. Kharkov, 1940.
4. Platonov, K.I. Psychotherapy. Kharkov: UPNI, 1930.
5. Platonov, K.I. Word as a Physiological and Therapeutic Factor. Second Edition. Moscow: Medgiz, 1957; Third Edition, 1961.
6. Platonov, K.I. On the Formation of the Combinative-Motor Reflex in Humans to Joint Sound and Light Stimuli: Dissertation for the Degree of Doctor of Medicine. Impe-

rial Military Medical Academy, St. Petersburg. Typ. of the Main Directorate of Edicts, 1912.

7. Praykin, V. Healing with Words. Trud, 1985, 14-09, 3.

8. Preisman, A.B. Hypnosis in the Practice of a Gynecologist. Ural Medical Journal, 1930, No. 1, pp. 52-54.

9. Raikov, V.L. The Influence of Deep Hypnosis on Reserve Memory Capabilities and Registration of the Hypnotic State Level Using EEG. Psychological Research in the Practice of a Medical Expert: Collection of Scientific Papers of the TSEITIN MSO RSFSR. Moscow, 1969. pp. 128-136.

10. Raikov, V.L. Study of the Somnambulistic Stage of Hypnosis with the Phenomenon of Induced Role During the Active Activity of the Hypnotized Subject. Therapy of Mental Disorders. Moscow: Medgiz, 1968. pp. 463-469.

11. Raikov, V.L. On the Possibility of Improving Memory in Hypnosis. New Research in Psychology. Moscow, 1976, No. 1 (14), pp. 15-18.

12. Raikov, V.L. On the Development of Abilities for Visual Creativity Using Hypnosis. Scientific Notes of Moscow State Pedagogical Institute named after V.I. Lenin. Moscow, 1969, No. 331. Psychological Problems of Youth. pp. 140-142.

13. Raikov, V.L. Experience of Treating Neurosis of Obsessive States by Modifying the Higher School of AT according to Schultz with the Use of Hypnosis in the Conditions of a Psychoneurological Dispensary. Therapy of Mental Disorders. Moscow: Medgiz, 1968. pp. 392-398.

14. Raikov, V.L., Adamenko, V.G. On the Objective Study of the Hypnotic State. Therapy of Mental Disorders. Moscow: Medgiz, 1968. pp. 457-463.

15. Rozhnov, V.E., Rozhnova, M. Hypnosis from Antiquity to the Present Day. Moscow: Sovetskaya Rossiya, 1987. 304 p.

16. Rozenbach, P. Hypnotism. Brockhaus and Efron Encyclopedic Dictionary: in 86 volumes. St. Petersburg, 1893. Vol. VIIIa. pp. 726-734.

17. Rout, B. The Language of Hypnosis. Moscow: Eksmo, 2002. 320 p.

18. Sas, Yu.V. Application of Suggestion in Obstetrics and Gynecology. Questions of Psychotherapy (Abstracts of Reports at the All-Union Conference on Psychotherapy, Moscow, June 27-30, 1966). Moscow, 1966. p. 166.

19. Safin, V.F. Experimental Study of Suggestibility. Scientific Notes of Moscow State Pedagogical Institute named after V.I. Lenin. Moscow, 1969, No. 331. Psychological Problems of Youth. pp. 62-67.

20. Teaching Seminar with Milton H. Erickson, M.D. Edited and Commented by Jeffrey K. Zeig; Translated by T.K. Kruglova. Moscow: Klass, 2003.

21. Sukhorukov, V.I. Treatment of Hypochondriacal States of Neurotic Origin with Complex Psychotherapeutic Massage in Hypnosis.

22. Questions of Psychiatry and Psychotherapy. Tambov, 1977. pp. 411-414.

23. Sukhorukov, V.I. Application of Massage in Hypnosis for the Treatment of Thoracic Radiculitis. Theses of Reports at the VI Congress of Neurologists and Psychiatrists of the Ukrainian SSR. Kharkov, 1978. pp. 227-228.

24. Waterfield, R. Hypnosis. Hidden Depths: The story of Hypnosis. AST, 2006. 477 p.

25. Waterfield, R. Self-Hypnosis. Hypnosis. Hidden Depths:

The story of Hypnosis. AST, 2006. pp. 442-444.

26. Fedunina, N.Yu. Franco-Russian Contacts in the Field of Hypnotism and Suggestion in the Late 19th and Early 20th Centuries. Methodology and History of Psychology. 2011. Vol. 6. Iss. 2. pp. 74-91.

27. Hayvens, R.A. The Wisdom of Milton Erickson: Textbook in the Specialty of Psychotherapy. Translated by A.S. Rigin; Edited by M.R. Ginzburg. Moscow: Klass, 1999.

28. Hailey, J. About Milton H. Erickson. Translated by V.M. Sarina, Yu.A. Khudokon. Moscow: Nezavisimaya firma Klass, 1998.

29. Hoke, R.R. Behavior in Hypnosis. Forty Studies that Changed Psychology. 5th International Edition. St. Petersburg: PRIME-EVROZNAK; Moscow: OLMA-Press, 2003. Ch. 2: Perception and Consciousness. pp. 82-91. (Psychology Best Project).

30. Sharko, Jean-Martin. Brockhaus and Efron Encyclopedic Dictionary: in 86 volumes. St. Petersburg, 1890-1907.

31. Shertok, L. Hypnosis. Translated from French. Moscow: Meditsina, 1992. 224 p.

32. Shertok, L. Hypnosis: Theory, Practice, and Technique. 1961.

33. Erickson, M. My Voice Will Stay with You: Milton Erickson's Teaching Stories. Translated from English by L. Hoffmann; edited and commented by S. Rozena. St. Petersburg: Peterburg-XXI vek, 1995.

34. Erickson, M. The Strategy of Psychotherapy: Selected Works. Authorized translation from English and edited by L.M. Shlionsky. St. Petersburg: Rech, 2002.

35. Erickson, M. Man from February: Hypnotherapy and Development of Self-Awareness. Translated from English

by E.L. Dlugach. Moscow: Nezavisimaya firma Klass, 1995.

36. Erickson, M., Rossi, E., Rossi, S. Hypnotic Realities: Induction of Clinical Hypnosis and Forms of Indirect Suggestion. Translated from English by M.A. Yakushina; edited by M.R. Ginzburg. Moscow: Klass, 2000.

37. Yapko, M. Hypnosis for the Psychotherapy of Depression. Moscow: Marketing, 2002. 247 p.

38. Bernheim, H. New Studies in Hypnotism. Translated from French by Sandor R.S. International University's Press, New York, 1980.

39. Bernheim, H. Suggestive Therapeutics: A Treatise on the Nature and Uses of Hypnotism. Translated from French by C.A. Herter. G.P. Putnam's Sons, New York, 1889.

40. Bowers, K.S. "Hypnosis and Healing." Australian Journal of Clinical & Experimental Hypnosis, Vol. 7, No. 3, November 1979, pp. 261-277.

41. Cedercreutz, C. "Hypnosis in Surgery." International Journal of Clinical and Experimental Hypnosis, Vol. 9, No. 3, 1961, pp. 93-95.

42. Collyer, R.H., M.D. Mysteries of the Vital Element in Connection with Dreams, Somnambulism, Trance, Anesthesia, Nervous Congestion, and Creative Function. Modern Spiritualism Explained. 2nd ed. London: Savill, Edwards and Co, Printers, 1871.

43. Edgette, J.H., Edgette, J.S. Handbook of Hypnotic Phenomena in Psychotherapy. Brunner/Mazel, 1995. 318 p.

44. Fredericks, L.E., Evans, F.J. The Use of Hypnosis in Surgery and Anesthesiology: Psychological Preparation of the Surgical Patient. Springfield, IL: Charles C Thomas, 2001.

45. Janet, P. L'Automatisme psychologique. 1889.

46. Jones, L., Othman, M., Dowswell, T., Alfirevic, Z., Gates, S., Newburn, M., Jordan, S., Lavender, T., Neilson, J.P. "Pain Management for Women in Labour: An Overview of Systematic Reviews." The Cochrane Library, Vol. 3, 2012.

47. Lockert, O. Hypnose: Évolution Humaine, Qualité de Vie, Santé. Paris: IFHE, 2013. 715 p.

48. Van Der Hart, O., Brown, P., Van Der Kolk, B.A. "Pierre Janet's Treatment of Post-traumatic Stress." Journal of Traumatic Stress, Vol. 2, No. 4, 1989.

49. Powell, R., Scott, N.W., Manyande, A., Bruce, J., Vogele, C., Byrne-Davis, L.M.T., Unsworth, M., Osmer, C., Johnston, M. "Psychological Preparation and Postoperative Outcomes for Adults Undergoing Surgery under General Anesthesia." Cochrane Database of Systematic Reviews, 2016.

50. Sampimon, R.L.H., Woodruff, M.F.A. "Some Observations Concerning the Use of Hypnosis as a Substitute for Anesthesia." The Medical Journal of Australia, 23 March 1946, pp. 393-395.

51. Wobst, A.H.K. "Hypnosis and Surgery: Past, Present, and Future." Anesthesia & Analgesia, Vol. 104, No. 5, May 2007, pp. 1199-1208.

52. Wolfart, K.C., Mesmer, F.A. Mesmerismus: Oder, System der Wechselwirkungen, Theorie und Anwendung des thierischen Magnetismus als die allgemeine Heilkunde zur Erhaltung des Menschen (in German, facsimile of the 1811 edition). Cambridge University Press, 2011. (Foreword.)

53. Yeates, L.B. "James Braid: Surgeon, Gentleman Scientist, and Hypnotist." Ph.D. Dissertation, School of History and Philosophy of Science, Faculty of Arts & Social Sciences,

University of New South Wales, January 2013.

About the Author

Dr. Artem Kudelia is a psychologist, therapist, and coach with extensive expertise in integrative approaches. He employs a wide range of therapeutic methods, including cognitive, behavioral, hypnotic, psychodynamic, transpersonal, systemic and other approaches.

By incorporating different perspectives and techniques, Artem aims to provide a holistic and personalized therapeutic experience. He understands that coaching, unlike therapy, focuses on supporting individuals without severe mental health issues in realizing their full potential and achieving success in various areas of life. His work is influenced by integral models of psychology, which encompass all quadrants and levels of human experience. Artem embraces a multidimensional view of human nature, considering biological, psychological, social, and spiritual aspects in his therapeutic interventions.

Subscribe to my newsletter:
✉ https://psychemaster.com/early-reader-signup

Also by Artem Kudelia PhD

This educational publication explores the fundamental approaches in psychotherapy. The **Psychology & Psychotherapy Theories & Practices Series** extensively covers the history of these approaches along with their theoretical and practical aspects. It can serve as a textbook for courses such as "Fundamentals of Psychotherapy", "Fundamentals of Psychological Counseling", and "Fundamentals of Hypnosis". It is intended for psychologists, medical professionals, psychology students, and readers with a wide range of interests.

Psychotherapy Fundamentals Complete Guide

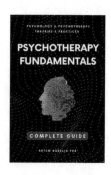

Do you want to understand the variety of methods of psychotherapy and choose the one that is best for you?

In the book, you will be able to delve deeper into the vast world of psycho-technologies and discover dozens of different schools of psychotherapy.

This comprehensive guide offering a unique exploration of various psychotherapy vectors that span the spectrum of personality theories and physiological concepts.

Gain a profound understanding of provocative therapy, humanistic therapy, somatic therapy, existential therapy, drama therapy, psychedelic and post-psychedelic therapy, anti-psychiatric therapy, and integrative therapy. Each chapter provides insights into the key themes and approaches of these psychotherapy vectors, expanding the possibilities for both practicing specialists and enthusiasts to enrich their therapeutic toolkit.

Seize this opportunity to deepen your understanding of psychotherapy, expand the horizons of your therapeutic work, and embark on a path of personal and professional growth.

**Hypnotherapy Fundamentals
Complete Guide**

Are you ready to uncover the secrets of hypnotherapy?

This comprehensive guide immerses you in the theory and history of hypnosis, providing a solid foundation for understanding the principles underlying hypnotherapy.

Explore the various techniques and approaches used in hypnotherapy training, including the art of suggestion and deepening hypnotic trance states, the creation of therapeutic propositions, and the utilization of the power of the subconscious mind.

Learn how to effectively apply hypnotherapy techniques to address a wide range of issues, from managing stress and anxiety to overcoming phobias and habits.

Gain an understanding of the transformative potential of hypnosis and its applications for personal growth and well-being.

Unlock the secrets of harnessing the power of the mind and creating positive changes in yourself and others.

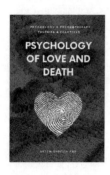

**Psychology of Love & Death
Therapeutic Path to Fundamental Balance in Life and Relationships**

How to Achieve Fundamental Balance in Life and Relationships?

Explore dualistic nature of human consciousness, along with the profound impact of seeking balance between fundamental continuums of **love and death**, **instinct and spirituality**, **masculinity and femininity** in shaping our experiences and relationships.

Explore the psychopathological profiles and manifestations of love and death, including profiles such as hysteria, paranoia, psychopathy, and others.

Uncover different types of love, from **eros** to **agape**, and study the **three-component Theory of Love**.

Familiarize yourself with **real-life psychotherapy cases** that illustrate the complexities of love, death, and therapy and gain **valuable insights** into the human experience and its challenges.

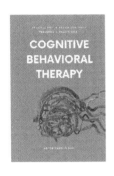

Cognitive Behavioral Therapy
Managing Anxiety and Depression

Explore the roots of anxiety and learn why it's a fundamental aspect of the human experience.

An in-depth exploration of **Panic Disorder**, addressing the irrational fears associated with it.

Examine the nuances of **Social Anxiety** and its impact on personal and professional spheres.

Dive into the world of **Obsessive-Compulsive Disorder**, unraveling its complexities.

Understand the genetic predispositions and learn effective strategies to manage obsessions and compulsions.

Explore **PTSD** from its roots to its biological manifestations. Delve into the trauma cycles, and discover therapeutic techniques for stabilization and overcoming trauma.

Grasp the degrees of **Depression**, from mild to severe, debunking common myths.

Breathwork Therapy Seminar Holotropic Journey to Unconscious Mind Secrets

Tap Into the Wisdom of Transpersonal Psychology!

This book is the <u>transcript of a seminar</u> that addresses the profound questions of **subconsciousness**, offering a unique perspective on personal growth and healing.

Gain profound insights into the workings of your mind and explore the mysteries of human consciousness.

Access practical exercises and techniques to facilitate personal growth, healing, and self-awareness.

Written for seekers of self-awareness, psychology enthusiasts, and anyone curious about the depths of the human mind.

Explore the integration of spirituality and psychology, uncovering your inner potential.

Psychotherapy
Introduction to Healing Vectors

Do you want to understand the variety of methods of psychotherapy and choose the one that is best for you?

In the vast world of psycho-technologies, there are numerous methods of psychotherapy that encompass a wide range of personality theories and concepts.

Drawing upon an integral framework, the book maps out the complex landscape of psychotherapy, encompassing vectors such as psychoanalytic, hypnotic, provocative, humanistic, behavioral, existential, transpersonal, cognitive, somatic, psychodramatic and psychedelic therapies, among many others.

This book will provide you with valuable knowledge that will allow you to choose the most suitable therapeutic path for specific circumstances and personality types.

Provocative Therapy
The Healing Power of Dark Humor

Who said that psychotherapy can't be hilar-iously funny?

Explore innovative ideas about the power of humor in psychotherapy and coaching.

Uncover the archetypal foundation of Provocative Therapy inspired by the myths of the Trickster and the Holy Fool.

Delve into the transformational potential of **Group Provocative Psychotherapy** and the important rules that define successful group dynamics.

Explore the effectiveness of **Provocative Coaching** and its focus points.

Dive into the fascinating world of **Provocative Drama** and its role in therapeutic interventions.

Explore the **pathopsychological profiles**, including **hysteroid, paranoid, psychopathic, obsessive-compulsive, schizoid, epileptoid, schizophrenic**, and **manic-depressive** profiles.

Humanistic Therapy
From Crisis to Self-Actualization

Do you want to explore a world where people are seen as unique holistic systems with infinite potential waiting to be discovered?

Immerse yourself in the theories and practices of humanistic therapy and explore the **transformative path from crisis to self-actualization**.

Unlike psychoanalysis, which focuses on internal complexes and personal traumas, humanistic therapy emphasizes the **study and development of positive personality qualities**.

Humanistic philosophy has also influenced fields such as **education**, promoting **empathy** and **support** as the foundation of learning.

This holistic approach recognizes the **interconnectedness of mind, body, and spirit** and seeks to stimulate personal **growth** and **well-being**.

Take the first step towards self-awareness, personal growth, and a more fulfilling existence.

Somatic Therapy
The Wisdom of the Body

Would you like to establish a connection with your body and access the source of wisdom?

Unleash the transformative power of **somatic therapy** and embark on a journey of **self-discovery** and **healing**.

Explore the profound connection between the **mind and body**.

Discover the **seven levels of muscular armor** and their connection to specific emotions such as sadness, anger, and fear.

By exploring different body segments, you will unlock **powerful techniques** for releasing pent-up emotions and promoting harmony throughout the organism. From **eye movements** and **jaw exercises** to **deep breathing** and **body movements**, this book offers **practical methods** for **accessing the wisdom of the body** and **restoring emotional balance**.

Acquire unique knowledge about **healing after birth trauma and psychosomatic medicine**.

Existential Therapy
Journey to Authenticity

Do you want to know who you really are?
What is your personal meaning of existence?

Embark on a **transformative journey** to uncover your **true essence** and embrace the **principles** of existential therapy.

Explore the rich philosophical roots of **existential psychotherapy** and find your path to **personal authenticity**.

Explore key themes such as **freedom, responsibility, meaning**, and **choice**, and learn to courageously and authentically navigate the complexities of existence.

This book provides **practical ideas and techniques** for **applying the principles of existential therapy** to your own life.

Gain a deep **understanding** of your **values, beliefs**, and **desires**, and learn to **embrace uncertainty** and **transform** life's **challenges** into **opportunities** for **growth** and **self-discovery**.

Drama Therapy
Potential of Psychodrama and Family Constellations

Explore the unique world of drama therapeutic approach!

Therapeutic model of intervention that encompasses **12 powerful speech patterns** capable of significantly **influencing conscious and unconscious processes**.

Through **psychodramatic techniques** and **family constellations**, you will **gain practical knowledge** to enhance your therapeutic practice.

Addressing a wide spectrum of **psychopathological profiles**, including **hysteria**, **paranoia**, and **obsessive-compulsive disorders**, this book equips you with effective dramatherapeutic activities and psychodynamic exercises.

It serves as a **comprehensive guide** to **crisis intervention**, **counseling theory**, and **strategies for addiction rehabilitation**.

Gain an understanding of the right hemisphere and the **neuroscience** underlying drama therapy, and learn to **navigate complex emotional situations** with **understanding** and **acceptance**.

Psychedelic Therapy
The Healing Power Therapeutic Journeys

Embark on a transformative journey into the world of psychedelic therapy!

Explore the fascinating **history** of **psychedelic substances** and potential benefits of working with consciousness-altering substances in clinical practice.

Learn comprehensive information on various **psychedelic therapies**, including **ketamine therapy**, **psilocybin**-assisted psychotherapy, **MDMA**-assisted psychotherapy, and **ibogaine** psychotherapy.

Gain knowledge about **mental health** in the **perinatal period**, the **role of hypnosis**, and the transformative power of **holotropic breathwork**.

Understand the profound impact of **psychedelic medicine** and the potential of **psilocybin microdosing**.

Explore the therapeutic applications of **ketamine** in the **treatment of depression** and **psychosynthesis in coaching**.

Beyond Psychiatry
Exploring Anti-Psychiatry Method

Challenge traditional psychiatry and psychotherapy!

This book presents an **alternative to conventional** ideas of normalcy and offers a **fresh perspective on psychological disorders**, inviting readers to question existing paradigms.

Delve deeper into **psychopathological profiles** and **anti-psychiatric** forms of psychotherapy, examining various profiles including **hysteria, paranoia, psychopathy**, and more.

Gain an understanding of the intersection of psychotherapy and existential philosophy, **challenging the myth of mental illness** within families.

Explore the **treatment of psychosis, trauma,** and **emotional disorders from a holistic perspective**.

Integrative Therapy
Personal Transformation Guide

Discover the Power of Integrative Therapy and Embark on a Journey of Personal Transformation!

This book challenges traditional divisions in **therapeutic approaches** and explores the potential of **combining multiple vectors** to create a **comprehensive and integrated therapeutic system**.

Immerse yourself in the world of neuro-linguistic programming (NLP), **cognitive styles**, **neurological levels**, and **integral philosophy**, among other concepts.

Explore practical methodologies such as shifting negative thinking, **creating rapport**, and using linguistic patterns to facilitate positive change.

Unlock the transformative **power of anchors**, **changing personal history** and submodalities.

Gain an understanding of maps of the world and the **metamodel** for **effective communication**.

Hypnotherapy Training
A Guide for Practicing Hypnotherapists

Uncover the secrets of hypnotherapy and improve your <u>practical hypnosis skills</u>!

This book explores techniques and practical skills for hypnotherapists.

Dive into the depths of the subconscious and discover the transformative potential of hypnotherapy.

Discover the benefits of this book, which delves into key topics and approaches in hypnotherapy training.

Explore developed techniques, including rapport-building practices and the use of matching postures, movements, and breathing with the client.

Unveil the levels of depth in hypnotic trance and the model of trance levels.

Engage in exercises that enable the attainment of different trance levels and explore the motives of trance and their application in psychotherapy.

Gain an understanding of different styles and orientations of hypnotic work, from hypnoanalytic and suggestive to behavioral and transpersonal.

Autism Family System Transformation Therapy Structure

How Do We Understand the <u>Hidden Causes</u> of <u>Autism</u> and <u>Possible Paths to Healing</u>?

Based on years of psychotherapeutic practice, the author presents a **unique perspective on Autism Spectrum Disorders** in this groundbreaking book.

Delve into the history and evolving **scientific** views on Autism, including Kanner and Asperger syndromes.

Gain valuable insights into the **psychological profile** of individuals with autism and learn how to **see the world through their eyes** by modeling their subjective experiences.

Discover the power of Integral Theory Quadrants and how they can form the foundation for effective **therapeutic approaches** for individuals on the autism spectrum.

Explore the **holistic** pathopsychological profiling of ASD, unraveling the fascinating world of savant syndrome.

Deepen your understanding of the **psychodynamics** of savant individuals with autism through **real-life clinical and practical examples**.

Unlock **alternative ways to communicate** and connect with individuals with autism, opening up new possibilities for interaction.

Investigate the interplay between **autism and evolutionary theories**, uncovering the evolutionary significance of autism and its relation to the unique strengths and challenges faced by individuals on the spectrum.

This comprehensive book goes further by offering an extensive **psychotherapeutic perspective**, focusing on the transformative power of **family therapy** (constellations therapy) and the **effective techniques** of Ericksonian therapy.

Authored by leading experts in the field, this invaluable resource provides reliable guidance for parents, psychologists, and therapists navigating the complexities of autism spectrum disorder.

Author Page

I would greatly appreciate it if you could take a moment to write a **review** and give a **5-star rating**.

Thank you in advance for your kind assistance and support!

Artem

Made in the USA
Middletown, DE
12 May 2024